S0-BRP-472

DR. RICHARD E. BUSCH III

Nationally Recognized Chiropractor

*SURGERY
NOT
INCLUDED

* DISCECTOMY
* FUSION
* LAMINECTOMY

FREEDOM FROM CHRONIC
NECK AND BACK PAIN

Copyright © 2020 by Dr. Richard E. Busch III

All rights reserved. This book may not be reproduced in whole or in part, by any means, without the written consent of the publisher. For permission requests, write to the publisher, addressed "Attention Permissions Coordinator" at the address below.

River City Books, LLC
PO Box 417
Raton, NM 87740

Disclaimers

*Surgery Not Included™ is not intended to diagnose or prescribe any treatment for any medical or psychological condition(s), nor are there any claims or offers to prevent, diagnose, treat, mitigate, or cure any medical or psychological conditions.

The book contains the ideas and opinions of its author and is intended solely to provide helpful information.

It is offered with the understanding that neither the author, nor the publisher, are engaged in rendering medical, health or any other kind of personal, professional services in the book. The reader should consult his or her own medical, health or other competent professional before adopting any of the suggestions in the book.

The author and publisher specifically disclaim all responsibility for any liability, loss, or risk, personal or otherwise, that is incurred as a consequence (directly or indirectly) of the use and application of any of the contents of this book.

The names of people mentioned in the case studies published within the book have been changed to protect patient privacy.

ACKNOWLEDGMENTS

I would like to thank the following who helped bring this book into being, or who encouraged me along the path toward helping patients recover without the need for surgery:

Dr. Richard E. Busch, Jr. and with a special tribute to my late mother, Jeannie Busch

Dr. John R. Ashton

Jaclyn Touzard, Editor of *The American Chiropractor* magazine

Elaine Fortmeyer

The American Chiropractor magazine

I would also like to extend a heartfelt thanks to my wonderful staff and my patients, past, present, and future.

DEDICATION

Surgery not Included is dedicated to my family:
Jennifer, my beautiful wife, and my children Elaina, Olivia, and
Richard IV.

FOREWORD
Foreword by Les Brown

Les Brown, the founder of Les Brown Enterprises, is the leading authority on releasing human potential and enhancing lives. As a renowned professional speaker, personal development coach, author and former television personality, Les Brown has risen to national and international prominence by capturing audiences with electrifying speeches, challenging them to live up to their greatness. "One of the most important things I've done in my life was to shake off mediocrity and continuously strive to live up to my potential greatness."

In my profession, I am very fortunate to meet and have a relationship with other professionals who are at the top of their industry and have lived up to their potential greatness. One such professional is Dr. Richard Busch who has dedicated his life to helping the sick and suffering.

"Applied knowledge is power. Because of the devastating impact that disease and sickness can bring into one's life, coupled with the astronomical cost of healthcare, people everywhere are seeking knowledge that can give them the power to improve and maintain optimal health and well-being."

Unfortunately, we live in a society where the response to illness in many cases, is to drug it out, burn it out or cut it out. In this groundbreaking book, *Surgery not Included*, compassionate doctor, dynamic speaker and insightful author Dr. Rick Busch addresses the agonizing and excruciating non-specific back and neck pain that affects millions of people.

Surgery not Included takes the reader on an all too familiar journey through the medical merry-go-round that includes endless testing, misdiagnosis and in most cases, ineffective and unnecessary surgery.

Committed to stopping this profit-driven, avoidable cycle of pain, drugs, and surgery, and in order provide hope for a better and more fulfilled life, Dr. Busch presents a cutting-edge integrated medical approach that will empower you to take control of your health.

The most compelling aspect of this book is Dr. Busch's focus on the whole patient. I've often said, "If you do not feel well, you cannot do well." Dr. Busch understands that back or neck pain affects not just your body but every aspect of your existence, including your job, your relationships and your quality of life. Understanding that pain is emotional and psychological, as well as physical, Dr. Busch seeks to heal his patients from the inside out.

Many people are convinced that their only choices are to live with chronic back pain or undergo invasive surgery and prolonged recovery. The idea that pain can be healed in a few short weeks with very little downtime seems too good to be true – but it is true. With more than a decade of experience combining the ideas of holistic health with technological advancements in the field of non-surgical pain relief, Dr. Busch has helped thousands of patients reclaim their lives – without surgery. In this eye-opening book, he uses real-life examples to illustrate the healing of patients from a variety of situations and with various medical conditions.

It is very difficult to write for both patients and doctors. Dr. Busch has found that fine line. He not only writes in a style that will intrigue doctors but through the use of simple language and diagrams, he allows the layperson to grasp the concepts as well.

As stated earlier, applied knowledge is power. While the information that Dr. Busch provides is invaluable, he also advises that patients must apply that knowledge by taking responsibility for their healthcare. They cannot expect healthcare professionals always to think of their best interests. Dr. Busch arms people with the tools and knowledge to be an informed participant in their recovery, letting them know they are not trapped between

Dr. Richard Busch III

their pain and surgery. The most important message you can gain out of this book is that you have options, there is a better way, but you must take action.

Underlying the medical information and practical advice, in this book is a road map that will give you the insight needed to reclaim your health and live a life of love, happiness, and comfort. Well done Dr. Busch - *Surgery not Included."*

LES BROWN

Les Brown Enterprises

CONTENTS

CHAPTER 1

Back Pain is Universal

CHAPTER 1
Back Pain is Universal

The American Chiropractic Association estimates that as many as 80% of Americans will experience back pain at some time in their lives,[1] and as many as 31 million are experiencing back pain at any one time. The numbers may seem astronomical, but the latest numbers from the Bureau of Labor Statistics report that back pain is responsible for 62% of people who miss work and account for 264 million workdays lost per year[2]. None of us has to look too far to find real-life examples of people with back or neck problems, and many of us have had personal experience.

Cumulative Pain

If you are over the age of 40, the likelihood that you will experience episodes of back pain is increasingly prevalent. You may have had a back or neck injury years or even decades ago, and at that time, it appeared to be asymptomatic or resolved. However, the condition may be cumulative as the damage to soft tissue and bone results in continuing degeneration, and the result is back or neck pain that can appear later in life.

A recent onset of pain can be confusing, as it may appear to have started from something as ordinary as stepping off a curb, sleeping in an awkward position, or playing a weekend game of touch football. This episode of pain is acute and sudden, but the underlying cause can be linked to the original injury or condition. Minor, intermittent episodes of pain have likely been occurring all along, yet they are not thought of as a chronic, ongoing condition, or related to the original injury.

Pain Does not Warrant Care

Many people live with chronic or ongoing pain because they do not perceive or consider their pain to be severe enough to warrant care. What they do not realize is that because the conditions or causes of their back or neck pain are cumulative, and more long-term damage may be incurred by not addressing their current symptoms. While the original injury may have seemed insignificant, the body compensates. Function is limited and continues to cause damage at the site of the injury. Many times, a disc condition may result.

How many family members and colleagues do you know who have had painful flare-ups years later that they credited to an "old football injury"? A chronic neck or back condition can develop years after a motor vehicle accident. In the meantime, the old injury may have been repeatedly aggravated, and the degenerative process keeps getting worse. Eventually, the cumulative cycle escalates to the point where it results in a disc-related condition, and the sufferer can no longer work and function normally.

It is common for pain sufferers to be unaware of the progression of their pain. Social or cultural attitudes and conditioning may cause people to deny or even hide their pain. An example of pain progression would be increased tingling or discomfort, or numbness, in the arms or legs. Living with a level of discomfort becomes "normal," and it may take a major increase in intensity or frequency of pain—changing from inconvenient pain to a loss of function, or from intermittent to constant pain—to cause someone to seek treatment. Since back pain and neck pain are subjective, many people who suffer will self-diagnose and self-medicate with over-the-counter (OTC) pain relievers that may help for a short time.

While OTC products may be generally safe and non-addictive, they do pose risks when taken incorrectly or over long periods. All medications have side effects, even OTC products. Eventually, the sufferer must talk to a doctor or make lifestyle modifications.

Problems with the Diagnosis

The origin of back and neck pain can be nonspecific. The spine is complex—composed of bones, nerves, ligaments, muscles, and cartilage—so the condition causing the pain can be difficult to pinpoint. A condition can create numerous symptoms and have the potential for a multitude of possible diagnoses. Often, it can be difficult for a patient to get a definitive diagnosis from the doctor about the source of pain.

In addition, there are varying terms or descriptions regarding spinal conditions, and there is a lack of uniformity among doctors when using medical terminology. Some terms that patients may hear from different doctors for the same condition are a pinched nerve, bulging disc, slipped disc, herniated disc, and ruptured disc. It is no wonder that a patient can be confused about a diagnosis and uncertain of the best treatment option.

As a chiropractor, I diagnose and treat patients who have chronic pain and severe disc conditions, such as herniated disc and degenerative disc disease, and their pain is interfering with their normal daily activities.

George, a 32-year-old construction worker, is an example of a patient who had chronic pain due to lumbar degenerative disc disease. George started having low back problems when he was ten. He was a typical kid who fell out of trees, fell off his bike, and played contact sports. All the injuries led to cumulative back problems that needed to be addressed and were causing problems later in his life. Throughout his adult life, he suffered from bouts of intermittent low back pain that he ignored the majority of the time, and he treated it with OTC products.

Periodically, when George's pain was severe enough, he sought chiropractic care, and it helped temporarily. However, he never achieved long-term relief because he never continued with the care. Then one day, when he was working at a construction site, he tried to lift a wooden-framed wall, and he was immobilized by excruciating leg and back pain.

For five long weeks, George suffered miserably, and he took large doses of OTC remedies. Finally, his wife, fed up with seeing him suffer, called a chiropractor. After three treatments, George was significantly worse. He was incapacitated. He could not even get out of bed to get to the bathroom.

When George's wife called my office, I recommended that they immediately call an ambulance and take him to an emergency room. At the hospital, George was sedated to enable the staff to perform an MRI. The hospital admitted George, and he was heavily medicated. He stayed for two days.

His diagnosis was torn hip ligaments and two herniated lumbar discs. The doctors told George that lumbar surgery was inevitable, but he refused because he had not been able to work for more than six weeks, and he could not tolerate months of recovery, physical therapy, and the loss of income.

The hospital released George, and he came to me for an evaluation. After an examination and review of the MRI films, I was confident George was a solid candidate for treatment with the nonsurgical DRS Protocol™. Within two days of beginning care, his pain had decreased significantly, and he was moving around without help. Within five weeks, George was back to work. Within eight weeks, he had a 100% resolution of pain.

Many people are fearful of surgery, and with good reason. A multitude of unknowns can occur when we choose to move forward with a surgical procedure. There are potential risks of scar tissue forming and from anesthesia, among many other risks. Anesthesia is of high concern for seniors. Until recently, it had not been widely noted that there is a significant danger, even when healthy senior patients undergo anesthesia.

After anesthesia, older patients can experience Post-Operative Cognitive Dysfunction (POCD). From the study, *An Update on Postoperative Cognitive Dysfunction*,[3] the statement and definition of POCD is as follows: "Postoperative cognitive dysfunction or [mental] decline (POCD) is increasingly recognized as a common phenomenon after major surgery. Because older age is a strong preoperative risk factor of POCD, the incidence of POCD is expected to increase as the population of older surgical patients grows."

Unfortunately, at times the impairments will be permanent, and the patient could continue to decline. Other patients at risk are those who have diabetes, Parkinson's and Alzheimer's.

Additionally, the potential for fracture, coma, paralysis, permanent nerve damage, and damage to the vertebrae exists, along with bleeding and clotting complications (many may be life-threatening or may require a blood transfusion), plus the MRSA bacteria and other contagious infections (that may require additional surgery).

Certain pre-existing diseases, medical conditions and bad habits—including diabetes, malnutrition, obesity, smoking, alcoholism, substance abuse, immune and connective tissue diseases, heart disease, kidney disease, cancer, depression, and high blood pressure—will increase the potential for failed surgery outcomes and complications.

A critical concern is that no one can guarantee a successful outcome from any surgery. Of course, there is always the possibility of death when any patient undergoes anesthesia.

Many patients I treat have had one or more failed back or neck surgeries. This problem is called failed back surgery syndrome (FBSS). By definition this is the continuation of the patient's chronic pain of the neck, back and or leg after surgery. The failure of surgery can be because of several reasons. Some are as follows: scar tissue, muscle stripping and nerve damage from retractors during open back surgery, and the reherniation of a disc(s).

These patients did not have pain relief, and in some cases, surgery made their conditions worse. Recent studies report that spinal fusion surgeries have only 38% improvement[4] and 40% will have a chance of having the same pain or worse. A notable number of these patients have had revision surgeries, and revisions surgeries have an even higher risk of failure. The likelihood of failure increases with each subsequent surgery.

Surgical outcomes are uncertain because the spine is complex. Surgery is a risky proposition because of the inherent risks of operations and complicating factors from pre-existing medical conditions. Also, there is a risk because of the close proximity of the discs to the spinal cord.

Residual effects can be scar tissue and nerve damage. It is for these reasons that no one can guarantee you will be pain-free or even experience significant long-term improvement from back or neck surgery.

At specific times surgery is indicated, and for some patients surgery will be successful. For others, it can have serious consequences and complications. Surgery should be the absolute last option. Once surgery is performed, it cannot be undone.

Some additional residual effects of spinal surgery can be as follows: numbness, tingling, change of gait due to muscle weakness, change of flexibility of the spine that will cause accelerated degeneration and can cause a higher rate of hip replacement complications,[5] even when the surgical procedure is considered a success.

Unless you have an emergency condition, it should be imperative that you explore every possible treatment option to avoid surgery for a spinal disc condition and allow your body to heal through noninvasive treatment methods such as the DRS Protocol™.

The Spine

Often people do not give serious thought to their spine, even though it provides numerous vital functions. The spine allows humans to stand in an upright position and gives the body a supportive framework.

One of its essential functions is to house and protect the spinal cord and nerve roots, which allow the brain to send and receive signals from all parts of the body, including the internal organs. The spine also provides flexibility. It is where muscles, ligaments, and tendons attach to anchor the arms and legs. This provides the ability to walk, stand, and hold the head upright.

The spinal column is composed of 24 stacked vertebrae or bone. Between each vertebra is a soft disc that acts like a small gel pillow, or a jelly doughnut. The discs function as shock absorbers that stop the vertebrae from bumping and rubbing against each other.

When you jump, fall, or walk, the discs absorb the shock and vibration, and they keep the vertebrae from jarring and causing damage to each other and your nervous system.

Ligaments, an essential part of the skeletal system, are strong, rubbery bands of connective tissue that hold the joints, bones, cartilage, and skeletal structures together and hold the discs in place. Ligaments flex, which allows bones their necessary movement but still enables them to maintain the structure of the skeleton.

Tendons are fibrous, inelastic bands of tissue that attach muscles to the bone. The spine also has joints, called facet joints, and they link and stabilize the vertebrae and allow them to move much like a knee or elbow.

Spinal Canal

In the following illustration, the arrow indicates the hole in the vertebra or the intervertebral canal. Each vertebra has a hole in the center, the intervertebral canal, that houses and protects the spinal cord. The spinal cord, a bundle of nerve fibers, is surrounded by tissue and fluid and is protected by vertebrae.

On each side of the spinal column, nerve bundles branch out in pairs of spinal nerves. Because of these nerves, a spinal injury can easily cause pain.

Spinal Canal
The arrow
illustrates the
hole in the
vertebra or the
intervertebral
canal.

When a doctor discusses back or neck pain, he or she will refer to four main spinal regions. One region is the cervical spine, consisting of seven vertebrae, which begins at the base of the skull and continues to the base of the neck. The adjacent region, the thoracic spine, consisting of 12 vertebrae, begins at the top of the shoulders and goes to the bottom of the rib cage. The next area is the lumbar spine, generally consisting of five vertebrae. Below that is the sacrum, more commonly referred to as the tail bone, which connects the spine to the pelvis.

Muscles are composed of both cells and fiber. The muscles next to the spine are the paraspinal muscles, and these run lengthwise along the spine. They attach to the vertebrae and support the spine. These muscles, when injured and strained, go into spasm to decrease movement, even if the injury is in another part of the spine.

When you understand how many structures the spine protects and the multiple functions it performs, it is easy to recognize the potential for frequent injury. Injuries can be due to accidents, overuse, abuse, and pushing the spine beyond its natural limits. The result is pain.

From Pain, Diagnosis, to Disappointment

Pain is our body's alarm system. It causes a protective reflex, and in the case of back or neck injury, pain may initiate "muscle guarding" to avoid further tissue or nerve damage. Pain will persist because of inflammation and irritation of the nerves.

Pain is a unique and personal experience. You cannot see the pain, you cannot smell the pain, and you cannot touch the pain. Pain can only be ranked by the patient reporting the pain on a scale. The scale ranges from zero to ten—zero signifies the absence of pain and ten is unbearable pain. You cannot see pain on an X-ray or through other diagnostic tests. Pain is not measured like weight or blood pressure. Although X-rays, blood samples, and other tests can detect problems that might cause it, pain cannot be seen.

Everyone experiences pain differently. How the brain interprets pain is subjective, and it is influenced by a multitude of emotional and physical factors such as the sufferer's personality, underlying health conditions, along with physical and genetic makeup, previous episodes of pain, preconceived ideas about pain, and the influence of drugs, whether prescription or recreational.

Because the causes of back and neck pain can be complex, in some cases, self-limiting or short-term, physicians are often reluctant to invest too much time into determining the source of the pain, and they often do not find anything specific in the initial examination. The diagnosis will likely be "nonspecific" pain. If an initial diagnosis of nonspecific back pain is given on the first visit, this may impede further diagnosing that could have been made through imaging or other diagnostic testing, unless the patient continues to complain.

There are standard guidelines developed for medical doctors that recommend they categorize patients with back pain into three general categories: nonspecific back pain, back pain that may be associated with spinal conditions, and back pain that may be associated with other causes such as cancer. The majority of patients—85%—fall into the first category.

The guidelines further recommend that physicians should not order imaging or other diagnostic tests such as MRIs or X-rays for nonspecific back pain patients. The guidelines recommend that those tests should be reserved for patients suspected of having more serious underlying conditions, such as infection or cancer. Paraphrasing a past president of the American Pain Society, who said, "The mystery begins with the first visit to the doctor and then continues from there since the exact cause of back pain is never found in 85% of patients."

As of early 2017, The American College of Physicians published their clinical practice guidelines saying that it is recommended to treat acute (sudden onset of back pain) or subacute (meaning back pain for a longer time) low back pain without drugs and to use therapies that include spinal manipulations, heat and massage among others. If patients continue to have pain, then take NSAIDs like ibuprofen. X-rays or MRIs are not likely to be ordered until a patient has had six weeks of conservative care.

Developing an accurate diagnosis for neck and back pain can be significantly more difficult than for many other medical conditions. The diagnoses of some conditions such as fractures, tumors, and pathology, are clear. However, many musculoskeletal conditions that have to do with muscles, bones, tendons, ligaments, joints, and cartilage, are considerably more difficult to diagnose. This is the reason I find it important to do a complete medical history, comprehensive exam, and X-rays or an MRI, if necessary.

The Disappointed Patient

It can be difficult for the patient who has already seen a doctor, followed the recommended course of treatment while being disappointed with the results, and perhaps even has been dismissed or put off by a doctor, to have the heart to listen yet to another doctor who supposedly has the answer. I have treated numerous patients who took a long time and went through much uncertainty before finally deciding to come to me for treatment.

One of the most memorable was Wes, who at the time was a 40-year-old engineer. Fifteen years before I saw Wes, he had fallen 25 feet down a manhole and seriously injured his back. Years later, he was still in significant pain, but his neurologist said there was no identifiable reason he should have any pain. Another specialist told him he had eight bulging discs, and he needed surgery. Prior to coming to me for an initial consultation, Wes was treated with three to four epidural injections a year since the time of his accident.

After evaluating Wes, I was absolutely convinced I could help him by treating with the DRS Protocol™. However, Wes had lived with his pain for so long and had been injected with so many epidurals that did not help, that the idea of a comfortable, easy, and pain-free treatment seemed too good to be true. Because of his treatment history, he was understandably skeptical of my recommendations. He honestly did not believe there was any procedure or treatment that could eliminate his pain, and that it would be without surgery.

Wes did not begin treatment right away. He continued treatment with a pain specialist, and he continued with injections in his lower back every three to six months. The pain relief was less effective with each injection. However, not long after my consultation with Wes, his wife came for a consultation and began treatment for a disc condition. Immediately, she had relief from the pain, and she was extremely pleased with her results.

A brief time later, Wes' mother-in-law started care for degenerative disc disease, and she had more than satisfactory results also. It was interesting that Wes would strongly encourage both of these important women in his life to undergo treatment with the DRS Protocol™. Apparently, he was not convinced that I could help him. Finally, Wes came for treatment, and within a few weeks he experienced tremendous relief and after completing care he was more physically active than ever.

It is very important for anyone with a severe disc condition - when given a choice between living with pain and enduring invasive and sometimes risky procedures - to research alternative procedures such as the DRS Protocol™. It is necessary to get a second nonsurgical opinion. I have helped thousands of patients understand that their lives do not have to remain limited by the painful aftereffects of spinal injuries or disease.

Even if patients have had previous back or neck surgeries and still experience pain, they can be helped. Most patients achieve significant changes within a few weeks, and the concept of a noninvasive pain-free treatment, the DRS Protocol™, certainly makes it worth investigating.

Throughout this book, I have included numerous cases from my practice, illustrating a variety and range of symptoms, injuries, and medical issues, to demonstrate that no matter what the situation, there can be hope. Pain need not remain an ever-present reality in your life. The choice to seek nonsurgical and noninvasive treatments is available. It is my hope that many will.

Back and Neck Pain Pipeline

Once back or neck pain begins to influence the choices of everyday life, the afflicted person normally sees the family doctor for a first level of care. I treat many patients who have followed a similar treatment pattern. I have since labeled this pattern the "back-and-neck pain pipeline." After that process has not succeeded in providing relief, many patients come to me to be evaluated for treatment with the DRS Protocol™. General practitioners are trained to look for the simplest explanation when confronted with a patient who reports having back pain. In the medical world, it is common to hear the phrase, "If you hear hoof beats, look for horses, not zebras."

In other words, they know that minor pain is often caused by temporary inflammation, and it may or may not clear up on its own, so they concentrate on treating the inflammation and pain rather than searching for the underlying source of the pain.

This usually results in the patient leaving with prescriptions for muscle relaxants, steroids, anti-seizure medications like Neurontin, and perhaps a few days of pain pills: Although, pain medications are now very restricted. This is merely the first step many patients take in their quest for help and pain relief. They often must convince their doctor that treatments are not working before they are considered to have a serious problem.

The next step of care is often physical therapy (PT). The patient has taken the medications, but they are not working. The doctor then may recommend four to six weeks of physical therapy in an attempt to promote healing, restore function, and just work the problem out. In the case of disc-related back or neck pain, there are two common outcomes of physical therapy; a patient will either have temporary relief, or the pain increases, and the patient drops out of therapy. Either way, the patient typically returns to the family doctor's office for the third stage.

At this time, the physician concedes that this is not the average, temporary, weekend-warrior pain, or that the patient is in the nonspecific back pain category. If the symptoms are chronic and severe, then the patient is now in a specialist's territory.

The general practitioner then refers the patient to a specialist, likely an orthopedic surgeon or a neurologist. The specialist will test, identify, and treat (it is hoped) the real cause of the pain. Since the obvious diagnoses—nonspecific back pain, strain or sprain—have already been eliminated, the specialist orders diagnostic imaging, which could include X-rays or magnetic resonance imaging (MRI). X-rays are useful in viewing skeletal structure and detecting breaks, bone disease, biomechanical alterations, and degenerative conditions.

An MRI creates a magnetic field around the body, sends radio waves through the body to detect changes in molecules, and creates pictorial slices of the body. An MRI is beneficial for viewing soft tissue such as nerves, muscles, ligaments, and organs, as well as bones. Both X-rays and MRIs are excellent tools for seeing the placement and alignment of the spine as well as the damage to the surrounding tissue. Another tool is the CAT scan (computerized axial tomography) or CT scan, which uses X-rays to create a comprehensive, computerized X-ray scan of an area rather than individual images.

Other diagnostic tests include electromyography or EMG. Needles are inserted directly into the muscles to test the electrical function of the muscles. Another test is nerve conduction velocity or NCV. During this test, electrodes are taped to the skin, and an uncomfortable shock is experienced. An NCV tests the electrical function of the nerves. The myelogram is a test in which a dye is injected into the spinal column, and it enables the doctor to see, via fluoroscopic X-rays, any bulge within the intervertebral canal that may be putting pressure on the spinal cord or spinal nerves.

A discogram is a study in which dye is injected into a specific disc to determine the integrity of the disc itself. A discogram is generally performed to confirm any internal tearing of the annulus (a disc wall). Many of these tests are frequently painful and can be expensive, and they are typically performed in a surgical setting.

A specialist, perhaps an orthopedist, will usually recommend temporarily treating the pain with epidural injections. There are over 9 million epidural injections performed each year in the U.S., and they aren't meant to be a long-term solution for back pain. Epidurals may help some patients with short-term pain relief and reduction of inflammation. They are performed in a surgical setting, and there may be a series of injections over time. Meanwhile, in many cases the patient continues taking medications like muscle relaxants and anti-inflammatories.

Epidurals are injections of medication made of a corticosteroid preparation and are placed directly into the epidural space in the spinal column. This is a similar type of injection many women receive during childbirth. However, the medications injected for back pain are different from those used for childbirth.

The injections can be painful and carry risks including ongoing headaches, nerve damage, and nausea, among other even more serious complications. Many research studies[6] conclude spinal injection therapy used for chronic low back pain has questionable outcomes. There is insufficient evidence to support the continuing use of injection therapy because there is a lack of research evidence. In addition, the FDA has issued a drug safety alert[7] and require a warning label for the epidural steroid injections which states: *Serious neurological events, some resulting in death, have been reported with epidural injections of corticosteroids. Specific events reported include, but not limited to, spinal cord infarction, paraplegia, quadriplegia, cortical blindness, and stroke.*

The warning continues with - the events happened with and without fluoroscopy and the safety and effectiveness of cortical steroids had not been approved for epidural injections. Injections may offer temporary relief, if any relief at all, but do not treat the condition causing the pain.

Surgical Procedures

If temporary procedures do not work, the usual next step is for the orthopedic surgeon or neurosurgeon to recommend surgery. Depending on the condition, the surgery type may be a discectomy, the discs protruding between the vertebrae are trimmed, or a fusion, the vertebrae are stabilized by being fused together using bone graft, metal rods and screws, or an newer alternative to a fusion, an artificial disc replacement (ADR) surgery. Surgery presents a host of risks, and the least serious one on the list is infection and the most serious is permanent disability or even death.

As reported in the article, "Alarming Escalation of Fusion Surgery – What Can be Done?", Dr. Ron Feise, states that spinal surgeries are performed in the United States at the highest rate of anywhere in the world. In fact, the surgical rate is nearly double that of other countries like Canada and Australia.[8]

Between 1993 and 2008, spinal surgeries performed in the US increased over 700 percent. It could be considered that access to care is easiest in the US, but that cannot account for fusions being performed at that rate of increase. Many experts state that as many as half of the fusions are not required, and they are performed on patients with diagnoses that should not be treated by spinal fusion.

Surgery will help some cases, although many of these surgeries will have short-term results, at best. Moreover, this may only be the beginning of a patient's journey in attempting to find help.

Periodically, I talk with a physiatrist, a medical doctor who specializes in physical medicine, and we have discussed the long-term outcomes of our patients. He had worked within an orthopedic group for years. During one conversation, he confided that he had left the group after a disagreement on the management of their patients.

The majority of their patients who had herniated or degenerative discs were operated on without exploring all of the conservative treatments available, and often, never considering any of them. He told me that, in his professional opinion, the problem was surgery.

Surgery may help a percentage of patients for the short-term, but it often creates long-term problems. For that reason, he decided to leave the group. I told him that with my treatment option, the DRS Protocol™, I have had a strong track record, even with patients who have had failed back and neck surgeries. He stopped and said, "Can you just imagine how great your success rates would be if these patients had never been operated on in the first place?"

Dr. Jim Weinstein, Director of Dartmouth Institute for Health Policy and Clinical Practice, states in an interview in *Prevention,* "We've found that geography is often destiny. It's not that the rates of disease are different, it's the way they're treated that's different — from prevention to diagnosis to long-term care."

Dr. Weinstein noted that the reason back surgery is recommended may be as simple as the geographical region where the patient lives. "Depending on where you live, your risk of getting a spinal fusion is much greater just based on your ZIP code." [9]

Statistics from Medicare data show there are specific areas in the United States that have considerably higher per capita rates of back surgery than others. In some areas, the rates are as much as 20% higher.

The conclusion is that this could be considered a "surgical signature", or practice style, even though there are medical guidelines for treatment of back pain, and the guidelines recommend conservative treatments be tried first. Surgery should be the very last option. However, many doctors don't follow the guidelines and refer their back pain patients to a surgeon.

Surgery may immediately relieve pain, but it is not the lasting solution that many think it is. Surgery can only provide relief if a patient is experiencing pain from direct pressure on a nerve, and it does not offer any improvement at all in many cases. There are no guarantees with surgery, and you can never have a surgery undone.

Once these measures are exhausted, often patients still have pain. They are frequently told that the only treatment available to them is to manage their pain through medications, nerve ablation (destroying the nerve), or even spinal cord stimulators. The doctors have exhausted all they know, and so they conclude that the patient must find a way to live with the pain.

At this point, a patient may be prescribed antidepressants, if the doctor feels the pain might be increasing due to emotional stress or depression, and because antidepressants have migrated into chronic pain treatment. Why they help with pain is not completely understood.

In theory, some antidepressants may alter chemicals in the brain and spinal cord and perhaps block the pain pathway. Not all antidepressants help, and there can easily be adverse side effects such as suicidal thoughts. Patients who take antidepressants need to have careful management.

I successfully treat many patients who have gone through part, or all, of this pain pipeline. Even if patients have had surgery with limited or no resolution of their symptoms, they can still experience improvement through the nonsurgical intervention of the DRS Protocol™.

It is estimated that Americans spend more than $100 billion[10] each year on back pain including direct costs such as medication and lost time away from work. The true cost to patients, besides the loss of income and money spent, is lost time and lost quality of life due to pain, poor outcomes, and the stress placed on them and their families.

The Real Causes of Back and Neck Pain

The causes of back and neck pain can be narrowed to four major categories. The most common are herniated or bulging discs and degenerative disc disease.

Discs are the soft pads of tissue that fit neatly between each vertebra and act as shock absorbers. These discs separate and protect the bones from clanking together or breaking under stress.

A disc is made of a fibrous outer layer, the annulus fibrosis, which surrounds a jelly-like center called the nucleus pulposus. Wear and tear over time, or a sudden fall, or other injuries can weaken or tear this outer layer and allow the soft jelly material of the disc to push out, causing a bulge that can press on the surrounding nerves. This problem is referred to as a bulging or herniated disc and causes pain or weakness in the patient.

Normal Vertebra and Disc C6-7 Disc Herniation

Another common cause of back and neck pain is degenerative disc disease. As with all parts of the body, the discs of the spine degenerate over time and lose some of their ability to absorb the normal stresses placed on the spine.

Because discs are avascular and do not have their own blood supply, they must rely on a process known as diffusion to receive the nutrients, water, and oxygen needed to remain healthy.

An impeded blood supply to the spine will reduce the amount of oxygen and nutrients that would normally be supplied to the discs, and the discs go into a state of dehydration or desiccation. Desiccation produces a low-grade, chronic inflammation, and this causes pressure on the delicate spinal nerves.

The area of the body controlled by a compressed nerve will begin to malfunction. Compressed nerves can cause numbness and tingling in the hands or feet or muscle weakness in the arms or legs.

Dr. Richard Busch III

If left untreated, nerve compression can cause substantial and perhaps permanent damage. Degenerative discs also will become much more susceptible to injury from physical stress and even day-to-day activities.

Degenerative Discs

L3-4
L4-5
L5-S1

Another very common cause of pain that is related to herniated or degenerated discs is sciatic pain, which refers to pain along the length of the sciatic nerve, the largest nerve in the body. The sciatic nerve branches off the spine at the pelvis and travels down each leg.

A problem at the root of this nerve, where the nerve exits the spine, may be felt along the entire length of the leg and can cause leg weakness. Sciatic pain can be severe and debilitating.

Patients often misinterpret this as a problem with their legs, when the primary cause is the result of a bulging disc compressing a nerve at the base of the spine. Sometimes, with severe inflammation, the pain will also be felt in the hips and buttocks.

Sciatic Pain Distribution Pattern

Many people over the age of 50 may experience spinal stenosis, which can be a part of the natural aging process. The spine changes with age and degenerates over time, which can— and will—cause pain. The spine protects the spinal cord by surrounding it with vertebrae and encasing it in spinal fluid.

However, when a disc bulges or the soft tissue around the spinal cord becomes inflamed, the soft tissue can push into the spinal canal thereby causing a narrowing, which results in a compression of the spinal cord.

Narrowing can also occur in the canals that branch off the spinal cord. While spinal stenosis is most often seen as a condition associated with aging, it can also occur in young people who have had a spinal injury or other abnormal narrowing of the spinal canal. Spinal stenosis is also caused by scar tissue from a previous back or neck surgery.

Diseases such as arthritis and scoliosis can cause spinal stenosis as well. It most often occurs in the lumbar spine, but can also occur in the cervical and thoracic spine. When nerves in the lower back (or lumbar spine region) are compressed, they may become inflamed, causing pain in the skin, buttocks, and legs.

Nerve Root Stenosis(narrowing)

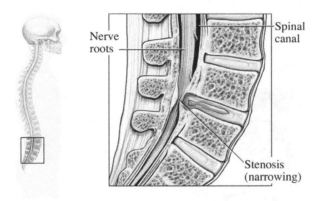

When you run your hand along your back, you will feel bony protrusions. These are known as spinous processes, and they serve as attachment points for the ligaments and tendons of muscles.

Facet joints at each segment of the spine add strength, flexibility, and integrity, as well as offer a range of defined movement (rotation, flexion, and extension) for each vertebral level. Facet joints are similar to other joints in the body, such as the knees and hips.

Facet joints work as a pair in the back of each vertebra. They link the vertebrae above and below, allowing movement of the spine, and are the areas where the vertebrae move and touch one another. If the very small amount of tissue between these facet joints, the articular cartilage of the joint capsule, becomes irritated, it can cause the same symptoms that are found with any other pinched nerve: pain, numbness, tingling, and a burning sensation in the spine.

Pain will often show up just in the low back or the buttocks, and this might be referred to as facet syndrome. Facet syndrome in the neck might cause headaches or shoulder pain.

In many cases, when doctors talk about arthritis of the spine, they are referring to the facet joints. These joints cause a patient who has arthritis in the neck to hear grinding when turning the head, this is due to the rough surfaces of the cartilage rubbing together. The grinding can be disturbing, and not to mention, painful.

Normal and Arthritic Degenerated Joint

There can be many other causes of back and neck pain, but I have listed the most frequent diagnoses that I treat in my practice. It is interesting that several of these common conditions are associated with age. It is extremely important to understand the cumulative effect that back pain will have in your life, even if you feel that it is "not that bad" right now. I see hundreds of patients every year who have waited until their pain became unbearable. Waiting is completely unnecessary when relief can be easily obtained.

The experience of going through the back-and-neck pain pipeline discourages many who seek relief for their pain but do not want to risk the consequences of surgery. Sometimes it is assumed that the majority of people seeking relief from back or neck pain are older, but this is an invalid assumption.

Back pain is the most frequent cause of inactivity in people younger than 45 years old. In fact, I treat many children and young people in their teens and twenties.

One such patient was a 16-year-old girl named Lacy. Lacy was a gymnast and cheerleader. One day in cheerleading practice, she landed hard on her backside. She developed back pain and had a hard time doing the normal acrobatic moves she had previously performed with ease. Lacy had some chiropractic care and saw an orthopedist. She was diagnosed with a herniated L5 disc in her lower back.

Lacy was treated with rounds of medication and physical therapy and received two epidural injections. The first injection helped for a short time; the second one made her worse. She could not sleep or lay down without discomfort. She was taking large doses of OTC anti-inflammatory medication just to get through the day.

Lacy's doctors told her that the only treatment course for improvement was surgery. However, surgery would have prevented her from participating in her normal activities for an extended period, and there was a high probability that she would never return to all of her previous pursuits.

Lacy's parents decided they wanted nonsurgical intervention before committing their daughter to the surgical path. Once surgery is done, it cannot be undone, and at the age of 16, there is a lifetime of consequences if it does not turn out well.

Lacy started treatment immediately, and within a few weeks, her pain had decreased considerably. Within only five weeks, she was back to her normal activity level, and surgery was not necessary. The body can heal itself, given the proper environment.

Dr. Richard Busch III

CHAPTER 2
The Painful Truth

CHAPTER 2
The Painful Truth

If you were to walk into a room filled with 100 people and ask how many are suffering or have suffered from back pain, the results might be shocking. Low back pain is the third most common reason for all physician visits in the United States, and joint pain is the second. We also know that approximately 50% of all United States workers admit to having back pain in the last year, and back pain is the most common reason for missing work.

As reported in the American Chiropractic Association's *Back Pain Facts and Statistics*, back pain accounts for then 264 million lost workdays in one year – that is two workdays for every full-time worker in the country. These are staggering numbers. Of those 100 people, there would be very few who had not experienced some degree of back pain.[1]

People often assume that back problems are the result of injury or some underlying chronic disease, such as cancer; this is rarely the case. Most back pain occurs in otherwise healthy people. A good example of this situation - a patient of mine named Pat - who was an otherwise very healthy person. Pat awoke one morning with numbness in her right arm. She knew something was seriously wrong and contacted her family doctor. She was given pain medication and told to return if there was no improvement.

By the next day, a nerve affecting her arm had become inflamed, and she was losing motor function. It was so bad that she could not hold a cup of coffee. By the middle of that night, the pain had intensified to the point that she went to the emergency room; there they administered an injection for the pain.

The next day, Pat had to be driven to her family doctor. The doctor told her that she had two slipped discs and surgery was her only option. At this point, Pat said she felt she was being rushed along an assembly line without knowing all the details, or understanding what was about to happen, or why she had no options other than surgery. She called my office in a panic while she was still sitting in her doctor's parking lot. She hoped I could help and that surgery would not be the inevitable decision.

After a thorough evaluation, I determined that she could be helped by my treatment, the DRS Protocol™. Pat's painful ordeal had already caused her to use all of her vacation time, and she had to begin short-term disability. Within a few weeks of starting treatment, Pat was able to return to work and soon was leading a pain-free life. I see patients just like Pat every day who desperately hope there is treatment for their pain. I am happy to tell them that there is.

We Live at Risk

The lifestyle of most Americans, as well as most people in the Western world, puts us at increased risk for back pain. Since the majority of back pain is not caused by trauma or disease, what are the real underlying risk factors?

The spine is often perceived to be just a bony structure that is impervious to the factors that affect our overall health, but this is not the reality. The structures of the spine are very sensitive to other health issues and respond to similar risk factors. For example, obesity is reaching epidemic proportions in our country, and the additional pounds affect the spine.

This can become apparent in a variety of ways, one of which is determined by where you carry the extra weight. If you carry the weight all in front, as many men do, it can increase the strain on the lower back and pull the vertebrae out of their normal alignment. This biomechanical change can mean that there is increased intradiscal pressure and joint movement, which can cause accelerated degeneration leading to chronic irritation and increased pressure on the nerves. Even if it does not cause pain, the increased pressure on the soft tissue structures (ligaments, discs, and nerves) can lead to the risk of severe injuries from everyday activities.

Poor dietary choices not only may cause obesity, but they can also cause deficiencies, imbalances, and inadequate digestion, which are major causes of health problems, including headaches, arthritis, and inflammation. Proper nutrition is imperative for maintaining the health of our bodies, and that includes the discs inside the spinal column. The medical community is acknowledging the connection between chronic diseases and diet:

"It is becoming increasingly apparent that chronic degenerative diseases (chronic inflammatory states) are evidence of food enzyme deficiency." The *1988 Surgeon General's Report on Health and Nutrition* stated unequivocally that "chronic degenerative diseases are dietarily related." (AutoIntoxication, by Dr. Howard Loomis, Jr.)

One of the most preventable risk factors is smoking. You may think it is ridiculous that smoking can affect the spine, but smoking decreases blood oxygen levels. The discs between the vertebrae of the spine and the nerves are not getting enough oxygen and nutrients to keep them healthy. Not only does this cause smokers to be more vulnerable to injury, but smoking also inhibits the healing process and can lead to chronic pain. Smokers are also more prone to disc problems as smoking leaches calcium from connective tissue such as cartilage, ligaments, muscles, and nerves—all of which make up a large part of the spine.

Studies have shown that smoking reduces the blood supply to bones. Nicotine slows the production of bone-forming cells (osteoblasts) and impairs the absorption of calcium. With less bone mineral, smokers develop fragile bones or osteoporosis.

Being a couch potato can also lead to back pain. If you lead a largely sedentary life, then you are not maintaining the strength of the bones and muscles in your back or neck. Studies involving astronauts following space missions show a decrease in weight-bearing activities diminishes bone density and muscle strength.

Even if a person has been active, if there has been a significant period of inactivity due to an injury or illness, it is advisable to ease into an exercise regimen. This includes warming up and stretching before activities.

Remember the Victorian-era old movies in which the grandmother was always harping about good posture? Well, she was right, especially in today's work environment, where employees often stay in one seated position for endless hours. Good posture can prevent a great deal of fatigue and strain on the spine. Poor posture can add strain and stress to the muscles and the spine.

The stress of poor posture can change the anatomical structure of the spine over time. This can constrict blood vessels and put pressure on nerves, as well as cause muscle spasms while contributing to disc and joint conditions. Many repetitive stress injuries could be prevented with good posture or the use of the widely available ergonomic office products.

Poor posture is a habit. I treat many patients who have continual neck or upper back pain that is associated with slumping over a desk, working on the computer, and being on the telephone for hours. This does not even begin to account for the role of stress in causing back or neck pain. It is vital to remember that straining and re-straining your spine, day after day, has a cumulative effect. Repeated strain can cause your posture to become worse over time and can lead to permanent damage.

According to the *Mayo Clinic Health Letter*, "Neck Solutions," 'Forward head posture (FHP) leads to long term muscle strain, disc herniations, arthritis, and pinched nerves. Other well-known effects of poor posture are headaches, mood problems, blood pressure problems, plus pulse and lung capacity problems. FHP is also known as the *texting disease*. We spend hours looking down at mobile technologies – iPads, games, E-readers, and cell phones.

Good posture improves our breathing, and good breathing improves the oxygen saturation in our blood. Maintaining good posture increases alertness, and we will feel better all day. Poor posture is a habit that is formed over time. One of the easiest ways to get into the habit of good posture while sitting at a desk is to use the trick of the old Victorian grandmother: balance a book on your head! This quick check will quickly show you how poor your posture actually is.

Fashion can also be detrimental to your spinal health. High-heeled shoes are popular with women, and it is doubtless they will always be popular. However, very high-heels that are worn every day force the lower spine into an awkward, unnatural position. High-heels slant the foot forward and bend the toes up. This causes the Achilles tendon to shorten, pushes the rump outward, compresses the lower back vertebrae, and causes muscle contractions.

While high heels may make the female legs and derrière look great, high-heeled shoes strain the spine with every step. High-heels are biomechanically and orthopedically unsafe. Occasionally wearing high-heeled shoes may not be damaging to the spine; it is the cumulative strain of regularly wearing high heels that cause the difficulty. Heels can create painful problems from the feet to the neck.

Flip-flops are a common sandal worn by all ages and genders. They are easy and perhaps comfortable, even though they offer limited cushioning, but flip-flops provide no foot or ankle support. You may have to curl your toes to keep the shoes on when walking or running, and your feet hit the ground differently. The lack of support and changes in gait can create pressure on the outside edge of the feet and less pressure on the heel; this, in turn, causes some rotation of the legs, changes to the angle of the pelvis, and creates twisting of low back. These and other mechanical changes can lead to foot, knee, hip, and back pain.

It is common to see adults carrying heavy purses or computer cases, and children toting heavy backpacks. People tend to carry too many items in totes, handbags, and briefcases, and they are unaware of the potential health risks associated with carrying excessive weight.

Carrying a bag that weighs more than 10% of your body weight will affect balance and posture. Extra weight is especially serious when the bag is carried over one shoulder. Any one-sided activity, including sitting on a wallet, or shifting your weight to view a poorly placed computer monitor, trains the body to become asymmetrical.

Any activity (such as carrying an infant on the hip) that causes a continual lean to the side, to counteract the weight, also causes the spine to curve in an unnatural manner. This causes the body to adapt its movement and stress the musculoskeletal system, which subsequently develops into premature joint wear and makes the spine more susceptible to injury.

We spend almost one-third of our day sleeping. Mattresses that are too hard or too soft can create unnatural sleeping positions and overextend the spine or not properly support the spine. If you have spent the night in a hotel or at the in-laws on a very soft mattress, then you know that the next morning, you probably will wake up stiff and feeling like a pretzel.

A medium mattress has enough "give" to allow the spine to be in a naturally-aligned position when lying on one side, but it also has enough support, so as not to give too much if you lie on your stomach.

Sleeping positions can help with back pain. Test sleeping on your side with legs drawn toward your chest, and place a pillow between your knees. Test sleeping on your back with your knees supported, and your legs elevated. These positions may also help for hip pain.

Sleeping positions are also a common cause of periodic neck pain and occasional headaches. Generally, it is better to use a pillow that does not force the head and neck position into an elevated angle. Feather pillows are preferred to extra-firm pillows because they easily conform to the shape of the neck. However, there are also excellent memory foam pillows available.

Another area of concern includes lifting and twisting. Few of us have been taught how to correctly lift objects. Even people who are required to lift heavy items at work often forget the rules for the safest way to lift once they are at home.

Contrary to a common assumption, you can cause strain or injury to your back, or even cause a serious disc problem, if you lift and twist when not in the correct position. Injuries can happen if you are doing repetitive lifting. Smaller items, such as bags of groceries, babies, lap dogs, and flowerpots can cause spinal strains, stretching or tearing of the ligaments, and herniated discs. This is because the person is often twisting and lifting from an awkward position.

Most people do not consider the implications of lifting while in an awkward position, or that there is a possibility that this could cause a severe problem. Even simple activities, done improperly, can cause spinal distortion and postural misalignment. Job duties that involve lifting, bending, or twisting will repeatedly strain the back. This is a common cause of ligament strain in the back, and even a simple sprain/strain may take months to heal.

Lifting should not be attempted when the knees are locked, because this forces the spine to do all the work, and the spine is not designed to lift heavy objects. I advise patients to "keep the shoulders over the hips and over the heels." It is critical to keep the back straight and lift with the knees to avoid straining the back. Never lift heavy objects without help.

It is interesting that many of the men I see have simply lifted something too large or too heavy for them. We have the perception that we are still 20 years old. As we age, we rarely consider that our muscles and ligaments may not be in the same shape as they once were. Even chores as common as gardening or movements as basic as getting up from the floor can cause strain and injury in different areas of the body. Use common sense; if it looks too big and feels too heavy to lift without help, it probably is. Get some help!

Chronic Illness

Chronic illnesses and long-term drug therapies inhibit the body's ability to heal. A limited healing capability can slow down and prevent recovery from back and neck pain and lead to a long-term condition. Diabetes impairs healing. Steroids inhibit all aspects of the healing process. Chemotherapy and immune suppression drugs also impair healing. There are many treatments and drugs too numerous to mention that can cause permanent changes to the cells, systems, and organs.

A good example was my patient Jake. He owned a trucking company and had type 1 diabetes. At 59, he suffered from both neck and lower back pain. He had previously had a cervical spine fusion because he had degenerative disc disease causing pain in his neck and arms. After the fusion surgery, he was still experiencing the same pain. He refused to have low back surgery because he was now very skeptical.

When Jake consulted with me, his chief complaint was pain in both legs. When he laid flat on his back, his legs would become numb and very stiff. He also had been diagnosed with diabetic neuropathy, which has symptoms of numbness and burning in the feet.

As anyone affected by diabetes, Jake needed to monitor his glucose level, follow a specific diet, exercise regularly for his condition, and take medication or injections. Since diabetes inhibits the body's ability to heal, treatment time with the DRS Protocol™ sometimes needs to be extended. Jake was treated with the DRS Protocol™, and his back pain improved by 90%. I told Jake, prior to treatment, that the numbness and burning in his feet might not respond to treatment because it was probably related to his diabetic condition of diabetic neuropathy. However, Jake's numbness and burning went away because his symptoms were related to pressure on nerves instead of his diabetes.

A longer than normal recuperation period may be necessary for anyone with a chronic illness or medical condition. Treatments for cancer may affect the rest of the body and its capacity to heal. Chemotherapy and radiation therapies cause chemical imbalances as they work to eradicate or control a specific condition or inhibit cellular proliferation. In innumerable cases, the treatment will destroy metabolic enzymes, and the immune function can be depleted.

When functions are depressed and enzymes destroyed, these can have additional adverse effects on health and the body. This imbalance may influence how successful treatment of the spine will be and affect the time it takes to heal since chemical imbalances slow down the body's response rates.

Living with Pain

No one wants to live with back or neck pain, but countless people do. The mere thought of having spinal surgery frightens patients, especially after they have experienced various ineffective or unsuccessful methods of treatment. Many more people in pain conclude the opposite thinking, "If I just have surgery, all my pain and suffering will be gone. I believe this because this is what I have been told by my doctor." They believe that surgery is the sole answer. However, there is no partial commitment to surgery.

Some patients believe there are only two options: pain or surgery. Therefore, in the past, many back-and-neck pain sufferers chose to continue dealing with pain medications and injections. Over time, these became less effective and had to be increased.

Now in the United States, the pendulum has swung to the opposite end of pain management. In an effort to abide with new laws and guidelines in place to stop drug abuse and addiction, many primary doctors will no longer prescribe opioids. If opioids are prescribed by primary doctors, the guidance for a doctor is to prescribe the lowest possible dose for 3-7 days.

Generally, the primary doctor will recommend the patient schedule with a pain management doctor, and the cycle may continue with injections, muscle relaxants, and anti-inflammatories. Many times, pain medications are not freely prescribed even by a pain specialist, and patients are prescribed non-opioid medications such as high-dose ibuprofen and drugs like Lyrica (pregabalin).

Lyrica is a drug developed for seizures and has migrated into the pain market primarily to treat, off label, neuropathic pain. Lyrica is another drug with potentially very serious side effects, and higher doses may be required overtime. Drugs like Lyrica are addictive and must be carefully monitored for abuse.

All doctors have to be very aware of patients who exhibit addictive or "drug seeking" tendencies because of the risk of abuse. The prescribing doctor has to determine the patient's motive and intent. Because pain is subjective and pain cannot be seen some determination has to be based on trust. The bottom line may be that some patients will have to live with pain, and they are told, "Not everyone gets well."

The recommendations for back or neck pain of anti-inflammatory medications, including nonsteroidal anti-inflammatories (NSAIDs) commonly cause side effects such as ulcers and bleeding in the stomach or intestinal tract. Additional side effects frequently experienced by patients on NSAIDs are nausea, vomiting, diarrhea, constipation, decreased appetite, rashes, dizziness, headaches, and drowsiness. These drugs may also cause fluid retention, leading to edema.

NSAIDs may increase the risk of potentially fatal heart attacks and strokes. The risk may increase with duration of use and in patients who have the additional risk factors of heart and blood vessel disease. Many NSAIDs and Cox 2 inhibitors like Celebrex and Meloxicam may cause secondary hypertension. Elderly patients are at greater risk for these side effects.

Types of Pain

Pain is conveyed to the brain by a type of sensory nerve that only carries pain sensations, and these extend to every part of the body. No matter what kind of pain is present in the body, both sensory and motor nerves are involved. This combination of nerve response allows the pinpointing of the location of the problem, how serious the problem might be, and the nature of the problem (for example, whether it is a burn or a sharp pain). Pain can have a number of causes. Pain is more than just an absolute sign of physical injury; it is also a subjective interpretation.

There are several different levels or types of pain. One way to determine the level of pain a patient is experiencing is by using the visual analog scale (VAS). The scale rates the severity of pain by starting at zero (0) for no pain, through ten (10) for unbearable pain.

Pain that is immediately disruptive to a normal routine is referred to as acute pain. Acute pain usually is a result of actual tissue damage, such as a cut, bruise, or a broken bone.

Other examples might include touching a hot object and burning your hand, catching your finger in a car door, or falling and scraping your knee on the pavement. Acute pain is a sudden and intense pain followed by an aching pain. It is typically short term and is resolved once the damage to the tissue is complete.

Dr. Richard Busch III

However, if the pain persists over time, it can evolve into chronic pain.

Acute pain can also be associated with poor circulation or dehydration that can produce headaches and muscle cramps. Acute pain will normally diminish as the area is treated and when the cause of the pain is removed or healed.

There is also a manifestation of pain known as referred pain patterns, which refers to pain that is conveyed by the internal organs and systems throughout the body to specific areas. A good example is pain felt in the left arm during a heart attack.

Because signals from several areas of the body often travel through the same nerve pathways in the spinal cord and brain, pain from a heart attack can be felt in the neck, jaws, arms, and abdomen. A gallbladder attack may be felt in the back of the right shoulder.

Chronic pain is generally defined as pain that lasts beyond the normal time to heal from an injury. This period is commonly thought of as four to six weeks, but some choose a period of two to three months. Chronic pain, pain that persists once the body has healed, can be categorized into two large groups.

The first group would include individuals who have a chronic disease such as osteoarthritis or degenerative disc disease. These people will have ongoing pain because their disease and degeneration continually progresses.

The second group includes those who have healed from the initial incident but are not fully relieved from pain. The pain continues for no apparent reason. This can occur for numerous reasons, including the fact that the body may have compensated for the injury and that compensation now causes more pain.

The body may have created scar tissue or adhesions, a natural mechanism for healing. However, the scar tissue itself may be pressing on nerves or within the scar tissue there may be trapped nerve fibers, and that is what is causing more pain. Chronic pain may also be the result of ongoing acute pain.

Long-term pain can also come from unknown causes, but this does not invalidate the patient's perception of pain. Pain occurs for a reason, and if it persists, there is a problem. One dilemma is not all patients with similar conditions develop chronic pain. It is not understood why some people develop chronic pain, and others do not.

Pain, from unknown causes that stimulates the nerves continually, if not resolved, can make the nerves even more sensitive to pain. This becomes a downward spiral for those with back or neck pain. Over time, there is so much stimulation of the nerve in the form of pain, that it changes the nerve and causes ongoing pain, even after the original problem has been resolved.

It seems that the pain signal continues to be sent to the nervous system, even without tissue damage. Also, there may not be a definitive point of pain. Perhaps the pain becomes the problem, as the nervous system is somehow misfiring and creating its own pain.

Neuropathic pain results from damage to, or dysfunction of, the peripheral or central nervous system, rather than stimulation of pain receptors. Diagnosis is suggested by pain that is out of proportion to tissue injury, and by dysesthesia (such as burning or tingling). In other words, rather than an injury causing pain, the nerves themselves are causing pain because they have become damaged and malfunction. The nerves become the source of the pain.

This category of pain can become a condition in which pain persists when there is no apparent physical reason, and it has only been recently investigated seriously. The patient may have developed an abnormal sensitivity to pain. This type of pain may indicate that the nerves carrying the pain signals to the brain may have been damaged from the previous injury.

These damaged nerves continue to broadcast messages of pain to the brain even though the tissue damage has healed. The pain feels very different from pain caused by tissue damage.

For many people, neuropathic pain feels like a severe shooting pain or a sharp stabbing pain. It can radiate down the limbs and cause pain along the entire nerve path. This pain is often chronic and continues for months or years.

One of the unfortunate outcomes of chronic pain can be depression. It is now widely understood that pain does not just include the physical sensation. There is also a psychological element to pain, that is why it can be so complicated and difficult to treat.

Pain affects the perception of the quality of life, which can lead to depression as the sufferer becomes frustrated and feels isolated by the inability to find relief — many people with chronic back pain report they feel worthless and hopeless because pain has majorly interfered with their lives.

Depression, fatigue, anxiety, anger, fear of additional injury, and stress or fear of losing a job are all chronic pain's emotional effects, and they interact in complex ways. Negative, emotional feelings even inhibit the body's production of natural painkillers and increase the production of a variety of chemicals that amplify pain.

The Harvard Mental Health Letter states, "People with chronic pain have three times the average risk of developing psychiatric symptoms—unusual mood or anxiety disorders—and depressed patients have three times the average risk of developing chronic pain."[2] As the pain increases and becomes the focus, the individual who is suffering may experience symptoms of depression and anxiety.

The body and mind are closely linked, and when pain is involved, it can be much like a vicious circle. When we experience pain, the body responds to a perceived level of pain. I treat patients who exhibit a remarkably high tolerance for pain; I am amazed to see how much pain certain patients can tolerate while other patients are in agony from what would appear to be a less significant problem.

This highlights why pain is so difficult to treat; there are no absolutes. Each perceives pain differently. There are no two patients, even if they appear to display the same exact findings on an MRI, X-ray, or other diagnostic tests, who will experience identical pain levels. Does this imply their pain is not real or is "all in their heads"? No, pain is a symptom of an underlying and sometimes serious condition, and it needs to be addressed. Unfortunately, many doctors may perceive certain patients' pain to be stress-related and treat the symptom as depression alone.

Pain not only affects the patient's life, but it also affects the lives of the patient's family members and friends as well. There have been cases where a patient has been in so much pain for so long that the family cannot remember what the patient acted like before the pain changed his or her personality. Sometimes, I tell a patient's spouse that I may even make the patient nicer because as the pain subsides, they are able to focus on a healthier and more active life.

Many patients are surprised by how quickly their lives return to normal once the pain in their back or neck has been addressed. Even if someone has lived with pain for years or even decades, they can gain substantial improvement of mobility and be free from much, if not all, of the pain and discomfort. Mark is a good example of a person who had long-term back pain.

Mark came to see me when he was 47. He was a dispatcher for a trucking company. His chief complaints were low back pain and weakness in and along the outside of his left thigh. Mark's pain had started intermittently about ten years earlier, but for the last five years, he had been in continuous pain, which had sharply escalated in the last four months. Mark's medical history was long and pockmarked with surgeries. Years before I saw him, Mark had a thoracic spine tumor removed when he was in his mid-twenties. This tumor was located on the vertebrae between the shoulder blades (T4-T7). Since the initial surgery, he had experienced weakness in his lower extremities and walked with a cane, as he had lost partial use of one leg. The weakness altered his biomechanics and caused him to have both hips replaced when he was in his late thirties. Mark had been through years of pain and suffering of varying degrees.

Mark had already had the usual "conservative treatments" with injections and physical therapy for his low back pain and weakness. He had been told by his orthopedist that he would need a lumbar spinal fusion. Mark was adamant about not having another surgery, but he needed help because he could not live with the level of pain he was experiencing.

After a thorough evaluation and examination, I concluded that the DRS Protocol™ would help Mark, with the understanding that the treatment period might be slightly extended due to his medical history. Mark's treatment proceeded cautiously so as not to aggravate any other medical problems. Mark had outstanding results: 100% resolution of pain. He was ecstatic. I treat him periodically to ensure he continues to maintain a pain-free life.

To all patients with previous complicating histories, I emphasize the need for a realistic expectation of their outcomes. It is not reasonable for patients to expect to see improvement beyond what their condition was 20 years ago. However, patients should expect to realize major improvement and pain relief.

Each patient is different, and treatment must be customized to the individual's situation. Even two people who are experiencing similar problems may require different treatments, and they cannot expect to have identical outcomes.

It is important to seek treatment at the onset of pain. When a patient has suffered from pain for a long period, there is the potential for permanent nerve damage. Pain itself is not cumulative, however, the condition that creates the pain may cause cumulative or ongoing irritation to the nerve, or the nervous system and that can cause permanent damage.

CHAPTER 3
The Patient Experience

CHAPTER 3

The Patient Experience

When I was close to graduating from Parker College of Chiropractic, I attended numerous advanced educational courses. During one course, I heard a presentation given by Dr. John Ashton about a new technology, axial decompression, which could nonsurgically treat severe and chronic lumbar disc conditions. He was extremely impressed with the excellent outcomes produced through this new technology when used to treat chronic disc conditions, such as herniated disc or degenerative disc disease.

At the time, Dr. Ashton told me that he believed axial decompression was going to become the future of treatment for chronic disc conditions. I felt he was right, and the thought of a treatment that would eliminate the need for surgery was exciting.

Axial decompression was developed by Allan E. Dyer, MD, Ph.D., who had served as Deputy Minister of Health in Ontario, Canada. The commercial name for the technology was VAX-D (vertebral axial decompression). Axial decompression, also known as spinal decompression, is a noninvasive treatment for chronic neck and back pain conditions like degenerative disc disease, herniated disc, and facet joint disease.

My original training is in chiropractic care, and since my family publishes the leading national chiropractic magazine, *The American Chiropractor*, I have had many wonderful opportunities to meet and interview some of the foremost experts in their fields.

One of those experts was Dr. Norman Shealy, a board-certified neurosurgeon, who is a nationally recognized author and founder of the Shealy Institute in Springfield, Missouri, one of the most respected pain management facilities in the world. Dr. Shealy developed the TENS unit (TENS is an acronym for transcutaneous electrical nerve stimulation). A TENS unit is a portable, pocket-sized, battery-operated device that sends electrical impulses through the skin to block pain signals. Dr. Shealy also developed the DRS table for spinal decompression (DRS is an acronym for decompression reduction and stabilization).

Dr. Ashton was involved in consulting on the development of this new system. It was used to increase the disc space between the vertebrae and relieve disc pain in the lumbar spine. The DRS System had some excellent new features that I favored over some of the limitations, at that time, of the forerunner, the VAX-D. These spinal decompression tables relieved low back pain by decompressing discs, relieving direct nerve pressure, improving the absorption of nutrients into the disc, and rehydrating discs, thereby helping to improve disc structure.

Nonsurgical spinal decompression evolved from traction. Traction is a method of stretching the spine, in an attempt to reduce back pain. Traction has been used for years in physical therapy. Various methods have been used in producing traction from motors to weights, to inversion or tilt tables. One of the limitations with traction is how the force is applied. Traditional traction keeps the spine elongated for extended periods and uses constant force that activates a muscle-guarding reflex, which creates muscle spasms.

However, spinal decompression provides controllable, distractive tensions to eliminate the muscle-guarding reflex. Because a logarithmic wave of distractive force, or the way the force is applied in spinal decompression, the treatment allows the application of a greater amount of distractive force to the spine, both lumbar and cervical, than traction, without the side effect of the muscle-guarding reflex.

The logarithmic application is important, as this allows spinal decompression to draw specific disc levels apart, which creates a negative pressure gradient from the inside to the outside of the disc. This allows the disc to be drawn back into its normal position.

When traction is applied, only the facet joints are drawn apart. Traction, over time, can increase the intradiscal pressure, rather than reduce the pressure. Potentially, this increased pressure can increase the patient's pain.

The significant lowering of the intradiscal pressure was confirmed in a study published in the *Journal of Neurosurgery*, authored by Drs. Ramos and Martin.[1] In this study, a cannula was inserted into the patient's lumbar disc space, and pressure transducers measured the pressure while the patient was treated on a VAX-D table.

A good visual of how a disc exerts pressure on the nerves is to think of a water balloon. If it is pressed on the top, the balloon expands equally on all sides beneath your hand. However, if it is then pressed on one side, the balloon bulges out to the other side. This is similar to how the disc behaves in the spine. Roll the balloon to the edge of a desk, and it bulges downward. This is how a disc can put pressure on the nerves of the spine. Remove the pressure from the balloon and the balloon returns to normal. This represents the decompression of the disc.

The amount of pressure that the disc exerts on the nerves is quite small. A study from Colorado University performed in the mid-nineties showed 10mm mercury of pressure on a nerve (the weight of a dime) would reduce the effective functionality of a nerve by more than 60%. This is not a lot of pressure.

I always tell my patients that I am not moving a refrigerator with spinal decompression. It is just making minor changes to the spine, but it is enough movement to improve blood flow, alleviate pain and inflammation, and help the body to heal.

I started using the DRS System, a spinal decompression table, in the first years of my practice. I saw the ability to provide relief and improve the lives of thousands of patients who were suffering from severe back, and now neck pain, and did not want surgery.

My practice was one of the earliest adopters of this treatment. I quickly learned that the manufacturers build great equipment but rarely understand how to integrate that equipment into an active practice. I further realized that this was such a new treatment technology that manufacturers did not comprehend the full potential of spinal decompression for positive, long-term treatment outcomes for severe and chronic disc conditions.

After treating patients with spinal decompression for just a short time, I began developing my own treatment protocol, the DRS Protocol™, which is customized for each patient's individual needs. The DRS Protocol™ incorporates spinal decompression, chiropractic treatment, and other important elements including exercise and nutrition.

The DRS Protocol™ manages the patient with specified treatment parameters, recorded benchmarking and tracking, reassessments and evaluations, and patient education. It is not limited to treatment on a spinal decompression table, but rather encompasses the complete patient experience. Treatment is specific to each patient's back or neck condition and is modified to fit the patient's individual needs.

My practice is located in Indiana, the heart of the Midwest. Historically, the Midwest is a very traditional and conservative area. This affects patients' attitudes toward traditional medicine. Spinal decompression was a new treatment idea, and at first, there was some hesitancy in the medical community concerning the successful nonsurgical treatment of severe disc conditions.

Success was rapid with the DRS Protocol™, and the word about this successful nonsurgical treatment got around to other doctors. Some doctors began to call my office to inquire about the treatment and how to utilize it. Since then, I have provided advisory work for some manufacturers, and I have authored several articles on the subject.

Some surgeons went so far as to say I was crazy for expecting success in treating disc conditions with the conservative, alternative care I was offering, even when their patients happily told them they had been successfully treated by me with DRS Protocol™.

Many patients readily understood the treatment concept, and spinal decompression easily made sense to them. Certain patients, such as engineers, farmers, and architects, completely understood the underlying concept, and while I treated them, they were trying to redesign some part of the equipment to enhance the appearance, structure, or even function.

After a few years, the proof was in the multitude of happy and satisfied patients who were able to live virtually pain-free without having to undergo any type of surgical or invasive treatment. It was not long before many medical doctors started referring their patients to my office first, rather than immediately to a surgeon. In some cases, the surgeons started sending patients to my office, and I was occasionally referred to as their friend. I was experiencing remarkable success rates with the DRS Protocol™. By this time, hundreds of patients had avoided surgery by being treated with the DRS Protocol™.

I had continued the discussion with Dr. Ashton about the future of spinal decompression. The potential for this treatment technology was tremendous. During the next few years, I had calls from doctors everywhere in the United States, asking for advice about treatment with spinal decompression. They had decompression tables in their offices, but could not determine how and when to use the treatment for maximum success.

Dr. Ashton and I decided to work together to share the DRS Protocol™ with other doctors, so that they could treat severe and chronic disc conditions, and to assure that they could achieve comparable results for their patients. Our consulting with medical doctors and chiropractors now helps patients all over the United States and certainly has reached more patients than I could ever treat in my personal practice. I have dedicated my life to helping as many patients as possible to avoid surgery and live pain-free lives.

Surgical Outcomes: Side Effects

There are unfortunate side effects for patients who have had surgery for disc conditions, especially fusion-type surgeries. These surgeries have a shelf life of two to five years, if even that, before the patient may begin to experience Failed Back Surgery Syndrome (FBSS). FBSS can occur because the bones or vertebrae are fused together, and the fused bones no longer move normally.

The fusion surgery causes more movement and force on the vertebral levels above and below the fused vertebrae, and that leads to degeneration or Adjacent Segment Disease. This creates more of the same problems in the areas adjacent to the fusion, and this could also require surgery.   Multiple studies confirm that less than five years after spinal fusion, the adjacent vertebrae have disc narrowing or degeneration.

Unfortunately, fusions are dramatically increasing. According to the data, the number of fusions performed is now higher than knee or hip replacements. Many experts question whether the benefits of fusions are really there. While the rapid increase of fusions might suggest fusions are effective procedures; fusions have increased the need for repeat or redo spinal surgery after the first spinal fusion. And, many patients are not pain-free after they have had a fusion. In fact, I see the people that are worse.

Leading surgeons are finally speaking out about back surgeries. Orthopedic surgeon Dr. Ralph Rashbaum, in an interview for *SpineUniverse.com*, had some compelling comments about back surgeries: "Most back surgeries are elective, and most patients 'chose' to have back surgery." When consulting with patients, Dr.

Rahsbaum asks them, "You know why they call it back surgery? Because you [will] keep coming back."

Again, Dr. Rahsbaum warns patients by telling them, "Your first surgery is usually just your first surgery. Over your lifetime, you will have more surgery, because that first surgery alters the mechanics of the spine, and it inevitably accelerates degeneration." Yes, there are serious reasons to have back surgery according to Rashbaum, but these account for about ten percent of spine surgeries; ninety percent is because "my back hurts."

Dr. Rashbaum advises that the best thing to do is not have spine surgery: "When in doubt about having back surgery, always get a second or even a third opinion before having surgery. [And] Always find out about alternative treatment options."

The risk of repeat surgery in the first years after a lumbar fusion surgery is high because the fusion itself increases the degeneration process because it stops movement and puts more stress above and below the fusion level.

For many years, studies have shown the poor long-term outcomes of spinal fusion, but many patients still believe that surgery will be a miracle cure. Unfortunately, surgery is not, which is why there has been so much research and so many clinical trials performed with replacement discs. Unfortunately, statistics show that that disc replacements surgeries have very similar outcomes as fusion surgeries.

It is well known that fusions are not a long-term cure and can cause many significant problems. In conversations with my patients, I have noticed that some surgeons are no longer rushing patients to surgery. What these surgeons are recommending is that patients wait until they can no longer bear the pain before even considering surgery.

Cindy - an actual neck pain patient and spine surgeon - called into the Diane Rehm Show as they were discussing the topic: "The Concerns about the Increase in Spinal Fusion", and said she had suffered from numbness in both hands and had to stop performing surgeries. Cindy had seen several neurosurgeons, and almost all had recommended a five-disc fusion for the bulging discs in her neck caused by an old whiplash injury. Cindy, the surgeon, told her doctors she absolutely had to look for an alternative treatment or, "This is going to ruin my career."

Cindy talked with one more neurosurgeon who recommended an alternative treatment therapy, nonsurgical spinal decompression. The neurosurgeon understood Cindy's fears. According to the Cindy, "I got rid of three bulging discs and [now] no pain, no tingling in my hand. I think a lot [of surgeons] aren't aware of alternative medicine's options."

After surgery for disc conditions of the back or neck, patients are often surprised and upset that they still have ongoing weakness and pain. The surgeon, Cindy, was concerned about this possibility. The problem is frequently due to scar tissue, which is fibrous connective tissue created by the body for wound repair. If the scar tissue forms near a nerve root, which is a common occurrence in back or neck surgeries, it can cause pain.

Nerve damage can be a direct result of scar tissue from the surgery. It happens to patients who have "successful" surgeries and yet continue to have pain. Reoccurrence of pain can happen most often about 6 to 12 weeks after the surgery and can follow an initial period of pain relief. The patient just slowly redevelops pain.

Even when a doctor says that scar tissue will be minimal, it can still be devastating, as it takes such a small amount of scar tissue to cause ongoing pain. Internal scar tissue can create adhesions and attach to internal structures causing pain. Scar tissue can be a debilitating side effect of surgery because it can wrap around a nerve and more-or-less strangle or compress it over time. The pain caused can vary from mild to extreme, and it can cause constant or intermittent numbness and low back pain that radiates into the legs. This is known as sciatica, which can come on slowly, leading to an increase in intensity, and can even lead to a loss of coordination and restricted movement. In the neck area, a similar occurrence can take place. Some of the symptoms are pain down the arm, a weak hand grip, and numbness.

When scar tissue becomes a problem stretching exercise may be recommended to attempt to reduce the pain of the scar tissue contraction. If this is not successful surgical laser procedures are recommended to remove the scar tissue, and this even happens after "successful" surgeries. Sometimes this needs to be redone every two to three years.

Remember, it takes a minute amount (10mm) of pressure on a nerve to cause pain. That is all the pressure required on the nerves in the spine to cause pain and reduce function. The problem of scar tissue contributes to "failed back surgery."

The issue of chronic pain associated with failed back surgery was reported as far back as 1981. In 1994, the publication *Spine* featured an article entitled, "Outcome of Lumbar Fusion in Washington State Workers' Compensation", which stated: 'Most patients reported that back pain (67.7%) was worse and overall quality of life (55.8%) was no better or worse than before surgery. Conclusions: Outcome of lumbar fusion performed on injured workers was worse than reported in published case series.'

A study published in *Orthopedics*, December 2015, Vol.38, 12, "Return to Work after Diskongenic Fusion in Workers' Compensation Subjects", reported that of the 1037 qualified patients with degenerative disc disease studied between 1993 and 2013, 76% never returned to work. And, the patients had acquired pain medication dependency, high rates of failed back surgery, and these patients required additional surgeries.

Given these facts and the fact that many other studies show that after disc surgeries pain can reoccur as often as 50%, the question is - why is surgery recommended so readily and so frequently. The short answer is surgeons perform surgery - that is what they do.

A surgeon is a highly trained doctor who has spent many years learning his or her craft and, by definition, specializes in the removal of organs, masses, and tumors, as well as other procedures using a scalpel. Surgeons also surgically treat disease, injury, and deformities. As a population, we could not live as long without them. They are trained in surgical intervention and have certainly performed many miraculous deeds.

A friend of mine, who is a surgeon, once told me that he had become tired of being ambushed by people at gatherings. They wanted to discuss their medical problems, which usually ranged from minor to severe aches and pains, colds, and various other ailments.

After growing very tired of being continually quizzed, he began to tell them the truth, and it stopped. When asked for his medical opinion, he would simply say, "I am a surgeon. That means that which I can't cut out, I do not know about." While it is a humorous story, it underscores the fact that surgeons are trained to treat surgically.

You may notice when you have an appointment with a medical doctor that he or she may do a very cursory examination, if any examination at all. In decades past, as much as 80% of the diagnosis was listening to the patient's history and examining the patient.

Now, many doctors rely much more on tests, such as MRIs, CT scans, X-rays, EMGs, and many others to develop a diagnosis. The reason is simple. Medical doctors, as part of insurance networks, tend to rush consultations as they are only reimbursed for a 15-minute consultation and exam. However, some hospitals ask their doctors to see patients every 11 minutes.

A recent 2018 study published in the *Journal of General Internal Medicine* found the average patient gets 11 seconds to say why they are seeing the doctor before he or she is interrupted by the doctor; women are interrupted more often than males according to the study.[2]

A typical first visit with a medical doctor concerning back pain, the patient may be prescribed medications: anti-inflammatories and muscle relaxants. If this doesn't resolve the patient's problems, on a following visit the doctor normally will recommend physical therapy. It isn't uncommon for a patient to wait some time, at least six weeks before having any imaging.

Testing has come a long way, and insurance companies require objective tests before they will pay for treatment, rather than relying on the doctor's opinion. However, with respect to back pain, MRIs may not be conclusive or may show false positives and negatives. Pain cannot be measured with a test.

Some patients can have a disc condition that may not be definitive or appears to be minor on an MRI, yet it is not evident enough to diagnose. Either the report then reads "normal study," or there is no clinical correlation between the films and the patient's complaint. However, if a complete exam were performed and the findings reviewed, there would be clear indicators that the patient does indeed have a disc-related condition.

A disc condition may not be visible on the MRI, perhaps because most MRIs are performed with the patient lying down, and there is no pressure on the disc causing the pain. At this point, the patient is often given a prescription for medications like oral steroids, gabapentin, or Neurontin, and again told to come back if the problem gets worse. This scenario could be avoided if the proper examination was performed even when MRI results are inconclusive. Orthopedic and neurological testing can detect and allow treatment of disc-related problems early enough to avoid or limit the severity of pain later.

Treatment and healthcare decisions must be based on accurate diagnosis, but there can be errors in MRIs. Research shows that the accuracy of MRIs in detecting lumbar disc herniation is not exactly reliable.[3] Studies report that approximately 30% of patients who were positive for a disc herniation on an MRI did not have a disc herniation which was only discovered during surgery. Another 33% of the patients who had a negative finding actually had a herniation, "The Accuracy of MRI in the Detection of Lumbar Disc Containment."[4]

Have you ever wondered why many doctors do not discuss vitamins, herbs, and other natural remedies, or complementary and alternative medical therapies, (CAM), before prescribing medications, even though many medications have well-known and even potentially dangerous side effects? One explanation is the philosophical difference.

Allopathic doctors are traditional Western medical doctors whose general philosophy is to treat with drugs and surgery. Medical doctors, unless they specialize in Complementary and Alternative Medicine, (CAM), have a small amount of training in nutrition and biological medicine. Most medical schools teach a limited amount on the benefits of nutrition, nutritional problems, and complementary therapies. Complementary therapies may have been previously discouraged by their medical boards as being nonconventional. However, in recent years that trend has been changing.

During their medical education and the many days medical doctors are in active practice, they are flooded with drug information. If allowed by the medical facility, drug representatives leave samples of the new X brand of antibiotic, pain medication, muscle relaxant, and antidepressant. The representative is hoping to create a stronger relationship with the doctor. This has to make the doctor wonder whether these drugs might be best for his or her patients.

A doctor would be concerned about the safety, efficacy, and cost of a new drug and its advantage over existing drugs. Researching the medical literature is required to compare the efficacy of the newer drugs to any of the older drugs on the market. This can be difficult because many studies for new drugs are only compared against a placebo and not an existing drug. There is an overwhelming amount of information for doctors to process, and because the pharmaceutical industry advertises directly to the consumer; consumer advertising creates a demand for their product from individuals who have no idea if the drug is best for their situation.

It is a big job for doctors to prescribe a drug, and the patient may influence some doctors' drug choices. Fortunately, now there are applications like EPOCRATES that can help doctors with information on disease, drugs and drug recommendations, and drug interactions.

Ever wonder why health conditions are called a disease or syndrome, such as Alzheimer's disease, acid reflux disease, and degenerative disc disease? Any malady that is labeled a condition, syndrome, disease, or any other medical term cannot be treated in any way that is not approved by the FDA. Since almost every condition is now being named a "disease," this allows the pharmaceutical companies to develop a new magic bullet as a treatment for each problem and prevents doctors from trying alternatives that might also work. The pharmaceutical companies are big businesses, and there was enough influence on doctors' preferences in prescribing to require legislation to stop improper influence on medical professionals.

The side effects of the influence of pharmaceutical companies on healthcare are a topic unto itself. However, patients need to become more inquisitive and take more responsibility for knowledge about their own care. Every adult who can read and has access to a library or the Internet should thoroughly research conditions, medications, possible treatment outcomes, and side effects. They should not simply assume that the first recommended avenue of care is the only choice.

Just thinking back about the surgeon, Cindy, who was mentioned earlier in the book, she had seen several neurosurgeons for numbness in her hands. The first recommendations were surgery. However Cindy, as a doctor, knew she had better do her research because her whole career was on the line if her surgical outcome was less than optimal. Cindy chose to treat with nonsurgical spinal decompression – an important part the DRS Protocol™. She is now pain-free and symptom-free! Researching, at the very least, will lead to more educated questions. A patient who questions a medical diagnosis or treatment is not an aggressive patient, but a smart patient.

For those who have health insurance, their coverage and choices will be limited to the description and terms of their policies. Older indemnity policies allowed more choice of providers and care. HMOs (health maintenance organizations) may cost less, but the patient's primary provider coordinates all care and imposes restrictions on the choice of doctors, facilities, and other ancillary care. The PPO (preferred provider organization) is an insurance organization in which member doctors and facilities work with a specific insurance company at negotiated, discounted payment rates. In a PPO you are not required to have a primary doctor, and you can see any healthcare professional without a referral.

There are also EPOs (exclusive provider organizations), and these are managed care plans where the patients are required to go to doctors and facilities in the plan's network, except for emergencies. There are also POS (point of service plans), and they are combining HMO and PPO features with more freedom to choose your healthcare provider.

Of course, there is government insurance, Medicare and Medicaid or versions of them; each with its own criteria, payment policies, and schedules. Doctors participating in insurance networks may find themselves in a quandary between what the best course of treatment for the patient is and what will insurance cover.

In 2003, health savings accounts (HSAs) were legislated as an alternative to traditional insurance, allowing you to save money tax-free in an account for future healthcare needs. You control how the money in the plan is spent on healthcare expenses. There are also Flexible Spending Accounts (FSA) and Health

Reimbursement Arrangements (HRA). Both help the patient control their healthcare choices.

Doctors have a small amount of time to diagnose a condition or disease, and they are reimbursed according to insurance guidelines. The insurance industry has a massive computer database of the standardized times allowed per patient per condition. Insurance companies reimburse according to the patient's diagnosis, objective data, and testing. Regardless of whether the patient is hard-of-hearing, using a walker, or in need of a translator, the doctor will only be reimbursed for the standardized time.

All doctors contracted with insurance networks have to demonstrate proof of a patient's problems to obtain insurance reimbursement. If a patient has a complaint, the doctor must offer a solution. Usually, in the medical community, the solution is in the form of drugs or surgery. The easiest solution for the doctor is to order less extensive exams and rely on lab and diagnostic tests. If all other treatments fail they then refer patients to specialists.

All doctors wish to provide quality care (why else would we have studied and trained for so many years?), but the system is not always conducive to prescribing fewer drugs and carrying out the least invasive procedures.

I am very pleased to have trained chiropractors and medical doctors from all over the United States in the treatment of back and neck conditions with the DRS Protocol™. This training offers doctors a treatment method for disc conditions that will provide a more complete understanding of the patient and his or her underlying condition. We can help patients with treatment and care without subjecting them to the potential side effects of drugs and surgery. And the results are replicable and amazing!

My principal desire for sharing my professional knowledge in *Surgery not Included* is to inform as many people as possible, including doctors, patients, and patients' loved ones about the

DRS Protocol™. Then all doctors who offer spinal decompression can utilize it to the highest level and achieve the best results. I have also developed the Busch Neuropathy Protocol™, and I will discuss this successful treatment in further detail later in the book.

Since 1996, and after having successfully treated thousands of patients, I am able to report that spinal decompression has been consistently effective. It works and is a vital part of treatment with the DRS Protocol™, and the outcomes of treating spinal disc conditions are even more predictable and the success rates even higher. I have dedicated my professional life as a Doctor of Chiropractic to treating a category of patients who would have had surgery or have had a failed back or neck surgery. The DRS Protocol™ with nonsurgical spinal decompression has been proven successful. It is steadily growing in public awareness and is here to stay. There are no side effects—except that the patient avoids surgery, ongoing pain, and job loss.

As with any treatment, a patient's lifestyle and bad habits may affect results. With the DRS Protocol™, patients can continue a normal life and have significant relief depending on their history, age, and other underlying health conditions. *Surgery not Included.*

Sharing this knowledge with both doctors and patients expands awareness of the option of an appropriate nonsurgical solution for low back and neck pain. The DRS Protocol™ can eliminate the need for surgery but still allows surgery to be an option in the future, if necessary. However, when surgery is performed, there can be side effects which can never be undone. They can include reactions to anesthesia that are especially dangerous for senior patients, unintended problems caused by the surgical "fix," or even naturally-occurring scar tissue.

My training is in chiropractic, which is the conservative management and treatment of health-related conditions and the human body. Nonsurgical spinal decompression melds with my healthcare philosophy and skill as a well-trained chiropractor.

When interference is removed from the nervous system, the function of the nervous system will be corrected, which will allow the body to heal itself naturally—given the appropriate conditions.

Prior to treatment with the DRS Protocol™, a patient may have considered other medical alternatives, including surgery. However, with the DRS Protocol™, we can provide predictable, successful outcomes for chronic disc-related conditions.

Some time ago, a friend's father was suffering badly from a chronic disc condition. I believed I could help the father through treatment with the DRS Protocol™. However, my friend's father had always taken conventional medical recommendations. He did not believe in alternative healthcare. Therefore, he just did not have the belief, or the understanding, of how the DRS Protocol™ could work for his condition.

This situation is very common and part of our human nature. We tend to gravitate toward that with which we are familiar, and we tend to take the word of people we consider to be experts, without question. What many people do not realize is that many common drugs came from nature.

For example, before people started using aspirin, they chewed willow bark or boiled it and drank the tea to relieve pain. About 400 BC, Hippocrates, the father of medicine, advised chewing willow bark to ease the pain of childbirth. For centuries, people all over the world knew of its power to treat headaches, fevers, and inflammation. They were familiar with this remedy and knew Hippocrates to be a great physician.

My friend's father had a conventional, medical mindset about surgery when the idea of treatment with the DRS Protocol™ was suggested. He was only familiar with traditional care, and he was not familiar with this treatment. The father believed surgery was his only option because doctors had told him so. He just wanted to get it over with, and to be free from pain.

I saw my friend two weeks later and inquired about his father. His dad had not made it through surgery. He died on the operating table. This was a very tragic and sobering outcome. While the risk of dying during surgery is small, there is still a risk—and it could be completely unnecessary. Sadly, he is not the only person that I know of who has had a similar outcome.

Unfortunately, many patients are only offered certain treatment options, according to their insurance guidelines. One example is a sheriff that I previously treated with the DRS Protocol™. He had two herniated discs, and I treated him with great success.

Several years later, I asked a mutual acquaintance how the sheriff was doing. I learned that he had re-injured his back in the line of duty. Since his injury was work-related, Workers' Compensation directed him to seek care exclusively within the medical profession. Certain states have strong preferences as to the direction of care and enforce these preferences if claims are to be easily paid.

The sheriff went through the treatments within the back-and neck pain pipeline, but he did not respond well to injections, pain medications, and physical therapy. Surgery was the next natural step and the preference of Workers' Compensation.

Within a week of his surgery, he developed a blood clot (embolism) that moved to his heart and lungs, and he died. Again, it is fairly rare, but blood clots can be a surgical side effect.

In addition to the risk of blood clots, anyone who undergoes surgery is also at risk from the dangers of general anesthesia. There are many dangers of anesthesia, including symptoms as mild as a headache or as severe as an allergy or stroke. The brain can be affected by a lack of oxygen delivery during surgery, and bacteria can be introduced into the innermost reaches of the body, causing infections that can be deadly. It is unfortunate, but anesthesia can also affect older peoples' minds and result in permanent dementia.

DRS Protocol™ Utilizing Spinal Decompression Is a Win-Win

The majority of patients that I treat have disc-related conditions. The noninvasive DRS Protocol™ utilizes spinal decompression to relieve pressure and allow the discs to receive the nourishment they need to heal. Treatment for patients with disc conditions will vary depending on their health plus the extent and severity of their problems. Even the most severe patients can be on their feet and back to work, within days. Surgery involves recovery time and medication, followed by physical therapy in some cases. In recent literature, it has been noted that physical therapy may benefit a post-surgical patient. However, it is not implemented enough. After surgery, there is significant downtime for patients, and it is often very difficult for patients to put their entire lives on hold.

The benefits of the DRS Protocol™, besides enabling patients to get better, are usually no downtime, no risk of anesthesia reaction and no risk of death. A recent study, "Influences of Spinal DecompressionTherapy", *J Phys Ther Sci 2015*, determines that statistically there is a significant decrease in pain and this therapy resolves problems with the disc.

It is important to understand that not addressing a disc problem can lead to other physical problems as well. When there is pressure on a nerve, feeling and strength will be affected, and function can be impaired. Pressure on a nerve can lead to visceral or organ related problems, as well. Many women currently on medication for intermittent incontinence may have a minor disc-related problem. This problem is so prevalent that a friend, who is a chiropractor, discusses having a practice that is dedicated solely to incontinence.

Unfortunately, women may just tolerate back pain and incontinence. They may be resigned to the fact that the cause is age or weight, and assume that it is not curable. However, if the problem is disc related, the DRS Protocol™ can improve their lives dramatically.

Another of the serious problems I treat is severe and debilitating headaches that limit patients' lives and stops them from being productive. Disc-related conditions in the neck may be the source of some headaches. Many patients may not realize that upper back or neck pain can be related to their headaches.

The term "cervicogenic headache" means that a headache originates from the cervical spine or neck. Every part of the body is connected to the brain by nerves. Pressure on a nerve close to the spine frequently causes problems in another area. In many cases, when a patient complains of pain or numbness in the arms, the pain may originate from a disc condition in the cervical spine or neck.

There are instances when a patient may have carpal tunnel symptoms in one or both hands, (carpal tunnel is the compression of a key nerve in the wrist, causing numbness and pain), but it originates from a disc problem in the cervical spine. Both this condition and headaches can be successfully treated with spinal decompression when they are disc-related.

Not being able to sleep is a frequent complaint of patients with disc conditions. They are constantly up and down all night or awakened by pain and unable to get comfortable. Many have to sleep in a recliner, on the couch, or propped-up on pillows. Many patients who are in pain are forced to sleep in specific positions, such as in a sitting or reclining position.

Some of my patients had not been able to sleep in the same bed with their spouses for years. They just put up with the pain because they did not want surgery. In addition, some medications can cause insomnia as a side effect. Besides insomnia, patients may suffer from anxiety due to persistent pain, and one problem will aggravate the other. This may hinder coping and lead to feelings of guilt. This is yet another reason why some patients are unable to rest peacefully.

The nervous system controls every other system in the body. It is the master system. Irritation and inflammation of nerves can affect one or more areas of the body and even hinder the function of the digestive or circulatory system. In fact, this can affect any system of the body and cause pain in any extremity. There are so many variables affecting symptoms, patients may have an endless list.

The Patient Experience

Patients who come to my office for the first time for treatment of back or neck pain may not know what to expect. To put my patients at ease, I explain to them that a complete medical history will be taken, a comprehensive examination will be performed, including orthopedic and neurological testing for clinical findings, and if they do not have current X-rays or MRIs available, then X-rays will be made.

Once I have completed the comprehensive evaluation, I sit down in conference with the patient and discuss my findings. When a patient is accepted for care, I discuss a definitive diagnosis, the term of treatment, and the expected outcome of the course of treatment. The majority of patients with back or neck problem will see tremendous improvement with the DRS Protocol™.

Each patient has a specific and customized treatment plan, and treatment will vary with the severity of his or her problem. Each patient's treatment is based on his or her medical history and condition. Relief of symptoms may be achieved easily for most patients within the first few visits.

However, some patients' conditions did not come about overnight. Whether their conditions are due to injury or degeneration, more treatment time may be required. Patients who are seeking a magic bullet are going to be disappointed because their expectations are not realistic. Treatment is a process.

With the DRS Protocol™, the average course of treatment ranges from four to eight weeks, depending on the diagnosis and medical history. Even the patient who may require longer treatment time is usually eager to do so when the cost of the DRS Protocol™ is compared to the cost of surgery—both financially and physically. There is the loss of time component when having surgery. Many times, a patient is not going to be able to work for weeks following surgery, excluding complications that could contribute to an even longer recovery. I am a firm believer in keeping people on their jobs whenever possible. The DRS Protocol™ is an excellent option with excellent outcomes.

Effective communication is a skill and is the key to patient confidence. Lack of clear communication can cause stress to the patient. A patient can be confused about the meaning of a diagnosis or treatment. My ability to communicate to a patient the meaning of the condition or diagnosis is a learned skill. My confidence in the DRS Protocol™ and discussing expected outcomes comes directly from successfully treating thousands of patients with chronic and severe disc conditions.

It is not unusual for a patient to start treatment being crabby. A few may be borderline belligerent at times. I understand pain can alter a person's personality, and I feel fortunate to be able to help a patient through the process. It takes someone who is trained and confident in patient care to see beyond words and actions and understand the underlying causes.

I treat patients who, because of their chronic pain, are difficult to deal with. Some feel their previous doctor discarded them; they had become high-strung due to pain. There is a small percentage of patients who cannot be helped by the DRS Protocol™. This may be due to other health issues or the fact that the patient's body may have a compromised ability to heal. If this becomes apparent, I discuss with the patient alternative conservative directions to pursue.

I stress that it is important to treat with an experienced doctor to achieve the highest success rates from spinal decompression with the DRS Protocol™. As you read the information presented here, I want you to know that there are successful alternatives to surgery. You do not have to live a life of pain.

When you finish this book, I believe you will have the knowledge to find a treatment that provides long-term relief, with a doctor who can deliver the best results.

CHAPTER 4
The Desperate Patient

CHAPTER 4
The Desperate Patient

Pain is a powerful influence on life and may cause people to do some interesting things. Patients struggling with chronic pain can have behavioral changes. Pain can cause people to say and do things out of the ordinary. Pain has the power to defy logic and override normal behavior. This may include taking large doses of over-the-counter (OTC) pain relievers. Because OTC products are familiar, it does not occur to the patient that they can be dangerous in large quantities.

Long-term use of NSAIDs (nonsteroidal anti-inflammatories) can stop the body from making prostaglandins. These are substances that help with some necessary physiologic functions. These include protecting the stomach lining and regulating blood pressure. Long-term use of acetaminophen can cause liver or kidney damage and has been shown, if taken long term, to increase the risk of heart attack, high blood pressure and stroke due to its toxicity.

Some patients may take OTC anti-inflammatories that contain the same active ingredients as other medications they take. This can cause an overdose even though the patient is taking the recommended dosage of each product. The FDA also reports that people who take NSAIDs and drink more than three alcoholic drinks per day can be at risk of gastrointestinal bleeding.

Some patients who are taking prescription pain medications report that they feel better when they take their pain medication and drink alcohol. This is a dangerous and deadly cocktail that most logical people would avoid. However, there are times that pain overcomes logic. Statistics from the Center for Disease Control show that between 1999 and 2016 overdose deaths have quadrupled and so had the sales of prescription painkillers.

Many patients rightfully do not want a surgical procedure but feel intimidated by or fearful of their doctor. In some situations, when a surgeon presses for a commitment to surgery, he or she can make a statement such as, "If we don't operate now, within a short time you will be in a wheelchair." I periodically hear reports of these types of comments from my patients.

Another frequent comment reported is, "If we do not operate now, you will just continue to have the same problem, and in a year you will be worse." No matter how insistent a doctor is, surgery may not be the only option, unless there is an emergency.

It is just as depressing for a patient who is told by a surgeon not to do anything until the pain is unbearable. Other patients live in a state of constant denial, ignoring the pain and refusing to do anything about it until they can no longer live with the pain. They are usually unaware that a nonsurgical treatment is available and would rather ignore their pain than face the prospect of surgery.

Antidepressants are frequently prescribed for patients suffering from back pain. This is because living with constant pain can create anxiety and depression. Once a patient admits or demonstrates depression, the doctor may believe that the depression is contributing to the pain.

One theory behind using antidepressants for the treatment of low back or neck pain is that low doses of tricyclic or tetracyclic antidepressant medicine may increase the level of certain chemicals in the brain, which can upset the chemical pathways for pain. Several studies show that while antidepressants may be beneficial for pain in the short-term, it is unclear how they work. They may also help patients sleep. The dark side of these medications, as with many pharmaceutical products, is that they have side effects that can be as mild as dry mouth or as serious as suicidal tendencies.

Pain often rules the lives of patients with disc conditions. Severe back or neck pain may limit the ability to do something as ordinary as picking up a glass of water, let alone working without pain. I treated a patient who reported that a surgeon who had evaluated him recommended a change of profession. A simple question: How easy is it for anyone to change a profession or career? Unfortunately, many people suffering from pain are forced to leave successful careers because they cannot perform the required duties.

If a patient cannot go shopping or enjoy outings to church or other activities, the result is a limited lifestyle. Social isolation and frustration may also result when physical activity is limited. It is difficult to know all the thoughts, fears, and perceptions at work in patients' heads. However, I do know that dealing with constant pain is fatiguing and mentally draining. Pain medications can cause drowsiness and result in severe fatigue along with the inability to perform normal activities.

At the beginning of care, I make a point of talking with a patient's spouse/partner. I often mention that I am going to make their spouse "nice" when we are all done with treatment. Many times, a spouse will look at me and say something to the effect of, "Well, if you can do that, Dr. Busch, any treatment would be worth it!" Invariably, while the patient is going through care, I have the opportunity to bring up the subject again and ask if the spouse is now nicer.

The common response is that the spouse is nicer than before and with less pain is able to get around to do things she or he has not been able to do in years. A problem with people suffering is they frequently make the people who care for them pay for their discomfort. Individuals in pain can be angry, withdrawn, and downright mean.

Pain can lead to resentment on the part of family and friends as well. It is very difficult to watch a loved one in pain, and as the patient's personality becomes more extreme as time passes, it can be difficult to understand.

Pain has the power to prevent people from socializing and establishing new relationships, and pain can damage existing relationships. Not only does pain create moodiness and emotional swings, but it can also limit activities and leave a spouse or partner to do things alone or suffer the same limited life. Pain can prevent a grandparent from picking up a grandchild. Older people feel stripped of dignity and lose the expectation of achieving a higher quality of life. Pain can control every aspect of a person's life.

Removing Pain

As a chiropractor, I deal with people who have varying degrees of disc conditions and levels of pain. Herniated discs, degenerative disc disease, and even stenosis cause pressure on the nerves and inflammation, and these are the cause of much of my patients' pain. In some cases, these conditions will respond to chiropractic care.

These problems are different than a subluxation, which is the imposition of bone putting pressure on a nerve and affecting the way that nerve functions. However, a condition resulting from pressure on the nerves from severely herniated or degenerative discs can be more difficult to treat. I treat these conditions with the DRS Protocol™.

Pressure on a nerve can affect the way any organ in the body works. This is demonstrated effectively with sexual dysfunction. Sometimes, the pressure on the nerves in the low back (L3-4) make it very difficult, if not impossible, for a male to achieve an erection or for a female to achieve an orgasm. This is because as the nerves exit the spine they are connected to an end organ. This end organ is innervated (connected to the nervous system by nerves) as are the muscles in the same area. If everything is communicating properly, organs function correctly. If there is a lack of communication between the brain and the body or organ due to pressure on the nerve, this can certainly affect the way organs function, as well as muscle strength and the sensation of the skin.

A patient came to me for evaluation. He had complaints about his back and some leg pain, and he brought an old MRI. After his examination and X-ray, I informed him that he had a herniated disc, and I discussed the possible outcome of treatment with the DRS Protocol™. Soon after beginning care, during a re-evaluation, the patient mentioned that his wife was very happy with his progress. Of course, I asked him why, and he said that prior to beginning care, and for the last several years, he had difficulty performing in the bedroom.

During his initial exam, he had never mentioned this as a problem, and he had never addressed his erectile dysfunction (ED) because he was embarrassed. He told me that after treating him for one week he noticed that the problem was resolved, and he was able to "perform" whenever desired. He and his wife were both elated with the results!

As intimacy decreases, relationships suffer. Many patients suffering from chronic pain perceive this as a lack or loss of personal control. Something that may also happen, because of a patient being in pain and feeling out of control, is the desire to take more control over other aspects of life. I frequently notice patients trying to control their children or spouse/partner as a result of their pain. It is a very complex situation, and every doctor should be aware of this possibility.

There are situations when patients may feel pain is helpful in their relationships. I recall a humorous story of my patient, Sandy, who was instructed to eliminate any activities that might aggravate or increase her low back pain. For two weeks, she was to discontinue activities such as raking, vacuuming, and bending to empty the dishwasher. A DRS assistant working with Sandy noted that close to end of her treatment Sandy was reporting 100% improvement. However, Sandy cautioned the assistant, "Shhh, I haven't told my husband that I can do any work like that." As far as her husband was concerned, it took quite some time for Sandy to return to normal activities.

The story about my next patient is quite the opposite. I had a memorable 86-years-young patient named Miss Betty who experienced a major flare-up as a result of a fall. She had a herniated disc that affected her so badly she was forced to use a wheelchair.

I did not know it until later, because of her dependence upon a wheelchair, she did not want to be seen in public using a cane, walker, or wheelchair. Betty gave me a hard time about getting her well again because she was not going to church until she was out of "that chair" and was not going to use the walker.

Her family wanted Betty to get a second opinion, so an orthopedic surgeon saw her when she was halfway through her care at my office. (Sometimes, improvement takes a little time if there's a chronic degenerative condition complicated by a herniated disc.) Her second opinion from the surgeon was that Betty required surgery. Betty said no, even though the doctor told her she would never be able to walk without a cane and she certainly was not going to be able to drive again. I treated Betty for many years with supportive care, and yes, she drove herself to my office, and she was walking without a cane.

Embarrassing problems that are usually associated with age, such as wheelchairs, canes, walkers, aches and pains, and problems with incontinence and impotence can contribute to patients feeling much older than they actually are. All of these problems can lead pain sufferers to believe that their lives have been destroyed. They cease to dream of getting better. They stop growing and developing and merely exist. For some patients, their pain becomes their identity.

We have all known people like this. Their whole life is framed in pain. Chronic pain is not a passive episode; instead, pain becomes life. It can be difficult for the people who are in pain to relate to others, especially if all the other people continually hear about is the account of pain, the doctor visits, and how awful life is. The people in pain may even have a feeling of grief about losing their former identity and life due to the pain. Moreover, while some may be relatively young, their lives have been fast-forwarded by decades. They may even be living as if death is imminent—when it is not. Life does not need to be this way.

Dealing with Doctors

Part of the frustration for patients is the experience of going through the back-and-neck pain pipeline. Even though I know many kind and capable doctors, the frustration is that patients have not only been told their only option is surgery, but they have already gone through the pipeline before. They know what the next step is. Everyone knows someone who has had surgery with less than a successful outcome. Invasive procedures carry their own side effects. I believe that if most people were knowledgeable about their treatment options, they would rather choose conservative care such as the DRS Protocol™.

Many patients are familiar with the idea behind chiropractic care and want an alternative treatment approach that provides the body with an environment to heal itself. However, I have seen patients who have not responded to previous chiropractic care and were told that surgery was their only option. Since they do not want surgery and they are not confident that chiropractic will help, they just get right back into the back-and-neck pain pipeline to try it again with medications, physical therapy, injections, and perhaps more extensive and painful diagnostic testing. Or alternatively they do not do anything. In many cases, they may feel misled and at a standstill.

Even after another round of unsuccessful treatment, patients are often told they still have a choice: they can have surgery, just as the surgeon had originally recommended, or they can choose not to have surgery—but they'll be back in this same place with these same choices, no matter what. At that point, they may be released to fend for themselves, or they may be sent for pain management and given continued medications and epidural injections. If necessary, they may have implantations of a spinal cord stimulator or a pain pump.

When patients decide against surgery, they can feel hurt and resentful if they have a sense that they are being talked down to by the physician. Patients are not ignorant for wanting conservative care. I believe that often the medical doctor does not understand the validity or efficacy of a conservative treatment such as the DRS Protocol™.

Because when doctors do not understand the alternatives, they do not recommend them, and many still are not aware of spinal decompression and the DRS Protocol™. Sometimes, surgeons intimate that the patient is not making an intelligent decision. That may end the decision-making cycle. The patient will break down and follow the surgeon's recommendation, even if they do not like the decision.

If the patient decides against surgery, or if the back or neck surgery fails, generally the next step will be a referral to a pain specialist. This is a medical doctor, who has acquired the necessary medical skills to evaluate and treat pain.

According to Orthopaedic surgeon, Ralph Rashbaum MD, who writes frequently about failed back surgery patients he sees: "We find out what went wrong. Typically, the patients I see clearly have failed back surgery syndrome (FBSS). They go back to their doctors [surgeons] only to find their doctors are totally disengaged in finding the truth. Unfortunately, this is common. An example of what a doctor [surgeon] may say to the patient is, 'I can't help you; you'll have to go someplace else.' This doesn't help the situation...these people become a referral base...in chronic pain syndrome in a pain doctor's clinic."

When a patient sees a pain specialist for failed back surgery, depending on the history of the patient, additional testing such as nerve functions tests and MRIs or X-rays may be ordered. If the patient has been to physical therapy prior, the next likely option of treatment offered would be epidural steroid injections. Injections are performed in a sterile setting, and the goal of the injection is to reduce pain through injecting an anti-inflammatory steroidal compound. These injections are not likely to offer long-term relief, if any relief at all. If some relief is achieved by the injections, then the patient is a candidate for more injections. Although, there are limits as to the number of injections that may be offered because steroidal injections have definite potential side effects.

When a patient is prescribed opioids he or she is required to sign a pain treatment contract which includes exact instructions: You agree you will not accept a prescription for pain medications from any other doctor, you will keep the medications safe, take the correct amount of the medication and not consume alcohol, not give to anyone your medication, file a police report if medication is stolen and always use the same pharmacy. There are a few other details in the contract such as agreeing to random drug screening. By not adhering to these major points listed, you will become a "past" patient.

In the recent past, pain specialists would usually prescribe pain medication, at times step up the dosage, or prescribe an even stronger medication to control the pain. However, guidelines have majorly changed and have become very restricted because of the opioid crisis, which is a complex and difficult problem. Some blame the pharmaceutical companies; some blame the doctors even though they were told that pain was categorized as the "fifth vital" sign by Joint Commission of Healthcare. In other words, reducing pain was good medicine. In 2001 doctors were actually encouraged to prescribe pain medication and assured addiction was not going to become a problem.

Some pain specialists prescribe the latest drug—not necessarily the best drug—or one that has not been studied for the patient's type of pain. Doctors may prescribe medications that are "off label," meaning they are used for a purpose for which the drug has not been studied or tested. In some cases, this may help the patient feel some better, but it is also possible that the patient will have an entirely different set of side effects and pain as a result. Unfortunately, many of these drugs are addictive and very powerful. They can alter the patient's personality and alter mental or physical function.

During surgery, nerves can be irritated, bumped, and stretched. Surgery can cause many unintended consequences such as long-term back pain, loss of movement or sensation in the legs or feet, loss of bowel and bladder function, and permanent spinal cord injury (although rare). Following surgery, patients are often angry with their doctor, even if they have a great doctor, because they may be worse due to scar tissue and possible nerve damage.

There are times when surgery is necessary, regardless of the inherent side effects. For instance, surgery is required immediately when a patient is diagnosed with Cauda Equina Syndrome (a condition where there is the loss of bowel control or bladder function accompanied by severe lower back and leg pain). However, those circumstances are rare. While the prevalence of surgery for moderate to severe disc-related conditions is very common, patients may have a much better outcome with noninvasive treatments such as the DRS Protocol™.

Almost everyone knows of someone who has had failed back or neck surgery, or whose outcome was not as successful as expected. One reason is the involvement of the nervous system. Spinal surgery is not the same as having a knee or hip replaced. With knee replacement, the normal expectation is to live a relatively pain-free life. Spinal nerves are highly integrated into the structure of the spine, and surgically altering the structure that protects and supports those nerves and the spinal cord can have a long-term and detrimental effect on the patient.

This is one of the critical reasons I feel it is absolutely necessary to perform a comprehensive physical exam and thorough case history, along with orthopedic and neurological exams. For those rare instances when surgery is necessary, it is imperative that I find this out immediately and that the patient knows as well. If it is the rare case I cannot treat, I immediately refer the patient to a specialist.

Conversely, for the many people with disc conditions that I can help, I want them to know that they do not have to face invasive intervention to find help and relief. They should know as soon as possible that they do have a successful alternative—*Surgery not Included.*

Patients with Health Issues

Many patients assume that treatment with the DRS Protocol™ is only appropriate if they are in otherwise excellent health. Fortunately, this is not true, and I have a great deal of success with patients who have a range of health issues. The following are some of the more common conditions that I see in my practice.

Osteoarthritis

Osteoarthritis, also known as DJD (degenerative joint disease), is a type of arthritis in which there is a breakdown and eventual loss of the cartilage between the joints. It does not happen overnight; it is a slow process of the cartilage breaking down. When arthritis occurs in the spine, it is called DDD (degenerative disc disease). The discs between the vertebrae degenerate and decrease the height of the discs. This can cause irritation and pressure on a nerve, resulting in pain, and can cause irritation to the facet joints on the backside of the spine as well.

The following are common symptoms: aching joints after physical activity, stiffness, and loss of flexibility after getting out of bed or sitting for long periods, and a crunching feeling or sound or a grinding sensation when a person turns the head or moves any other joint.

This type of arthritis is the most common, affecting more than 20 million people in the United States. Osteoarthritis becomes more common with age. By age 65, 50% of the population has evidence of osteoarthritis, and it tends to affect more women than men. A genetic component contributes to some cases. Other factors are obesity, poor nutrition, lack of exercise, changes in posture, and disease. I see many patients with this condition, and as the baby boomers age and obesity increases, I expect to see many more. Osteoarthritis can also be the result of an old injury that caused damage to a joint or the joint capsule. Over time, this can create a change in the movement of the joint and damage the bone around the joint.

Osteoarthritis can also result from improper movement of a joint over many years. The improper movement continues to put abnormal stress on the joint, and that leads to degeneration.

Osteoporosis

Osteoporosis is a condition of decreased bone mass, which leads to the risk of fracture due to the fragility of the bones. Anyone can develop this disorder, but it is more common in older women. As many as half of all women over 50, and a quarter of all men in that same age bracket, will break a bone due to osteoporosis.

The latest information regarding osteoporosis is that there is no single cause, but some causes are heredity, ethnicity, lifestyle, side effects of disease, and medication. Certain medications, including steroids such as prednisone, a corticosteroid, inhibit absorption of calcium in the intestine. Immunosuppressant drugs may also cause bone loss.

Due to the inherent problems associated with this disorder, a doctor must be aware of the patient's bone density during treatment. Bone density is checked through a Dexa scan that gives a risk score. As the disease progresses, a person's bones are very fragile and very susceptible to compression fractures in the thoracic and lumbar spine as well as the hips. In advanced stages, simple bending can cause a compression fracture.

The DRS Protocol™ is very gentle, and an osteoporotic patient can achieve good results and substantial pain reduction. This type of patient is closely monitored and has frequent re-evaluations.

Diabetes

Very simply, diabetes is a disease characterized by high blood sugar. There are two major types of the disease. Type 1 diabetes is usually diagnosed in children and young adults. It was previously known as juvenile diabetes. Type 1 diabetes is an autoimmune condition. The body does not produce insulin, which is a hormone that is required to convert sugar (glucose), starches, and other food into energy. The result is high blood sugar, which at abnormally high levels over time can damage tissue and organs and even cause death if left untreated.

Type 2 diabetes is the most common form. With Type 2, either the body does not produce sufficient insulin, or the cells do not recognize the insulin. Type 2 causes glucose to build up in the blood instead of going into cells. This can cause two problems: cells will be starved for energy, and over time, high blood glucose levels may damage the eyes, kidneys, nerves, or heart.

It is essential to know the extent of a patient's diabetes and to know how well it has been controlled before treatment. Many patients are able to manage diabetes by simply following a diet and by exercising. Other patients affected by diabetes require daily medication, along with dietary and exercise recommendations, and others require insulin.

Diabetes suppresses the immune system, slows healing, and can directly affect the nerves. Patients with diabetes may feel numbness, burning, and pain in their extremities due to a condition called diabetic neuropathy. Diabetic neuropathy is a common complication. The symptoms can have a range of manifestations, including almost no symptoms at all.

However, the symptoms can also be quite severe and include tingling and numbness in the extremities, weakness and wasting of the muscles in the hands and feet, problems with urination, and gastrointestinal problems.

Diabetic neuropathy is nerve damage resulting from high blood glucose levels and low oxygen levels, and this will be discussed in detail in Chapter 7. Another factor is the length of time the glucose levels have been affecting the nerves. Over time, the damage will increase.

Problems can occur in every system, including the digestive tract, heart, and sex organs. When treating patients who have diabetic neuropathy, it is important to differentiate between the disease process and a disc-related condition. Distinction can be very difficult. When a diabetic patient presents with a neuropathic condition, the exam findings may include diminished sensitivity plus complaints of numbness and tingling and burning.

Diabetic neuropathy will not respond to treatment with the DRS Protocol™ alone. Because people affected by diabetes have a suppressed immune system, this also means that the patient may not respond as quickly to treatment. Therefore, I discuss these limitations with patients affected by diabetes. Having said that, most will have great results from the DRS Protocol™. Treatment for symptoms of diabetic neuropathy will be discussed in Chapter 7.

With surgery, there is evidence that diabetics may have more complications than other patients following a lumbar fusion. The next story is a particularly memorable one of a discouraged patient with diabetes.

John was a 58-year-old with diabetes, and he was on a downward spiral. He had not monitored his diabetes closely, and he certainly did not watch his diet. While his diabetes was under control to a degree, he was not in good condition.

John was 75 pounds overweight, and he had been in pain with a lumbar disc condition for ten years. He was suffering from low back pain along with pain in his legs and feet. Diabetic neuropathy contributed to his foot pain. He was cantankerous and appeared to have given up hope.

As I talked with John about his diabetes and treatment for his disc condition, I impressed upon him the point that treatment would progress much faster and he would have the best results if he took better care of himself. With an eye roll and a shrug, (it is difficult to exercise when you have back, leg, and foot pain), John agreed to try to take better care of himself, and then he started treatment with the DRS Protocol™.

Within two weeks, John was feeling noticeably better. His low back pain was diminished, and his leg and foot pain were almost resolved! It was not diabetic neuropathy affecting his feet after all. The improvement gave John a lot of hope. He told me that because his foot pain was almost gone, he was excited. He really did feel like taking better care of himself. Before treatment with the DRS Protocol™, he did not see any benefit in watching his weight or his diet, since he was in pain all the time anyway. It took some improvement and a reasonable effort on his part, to convince him to continue with healthier habits. Then his improvement accelerated.

Patients living with chronic conditions may not believe there is hope for improvement. However, relieving the pain caused by their disc conditions can be a reality and can change their lives.

Heart-Related Conditions

Heart conditions include coronary heart disease, arrhythmia, heart valve disease, cardiomyopathy, and aorta problems. Many heart conditions can lead to heart attack and stroke. I have treated many individuals who have had heart-related conditions.

Patients who have had heart attacks usually have no issues at all in undertaking treatment with the DRS Protocol™, though a heart attack can cause extensive damage to the heart muscle and leave the patient with general weakness.

The DRS Protocol™ can help with reducing pain and alleviating weakness due to pressure on the nerves of the spine. Of course, any general weakness brought on by damage from a heart attack will not be improved.

Many heart attack patients who have blockages in the arteries will have stents surgically placed to improve blood flow to the heart. A stent is a wire mesh tube that is implanted in an artery using an angioplasty procedure. Stents are inserted through an artery, and this incision must be allowed to heal at least five days prior to treating with spinal decompression. These patients will achieve very good results with the DRS Protocol™.

In the United States, strokes are the number one cause of disability and the third most common cause of death in adults. Strokes are associated with excessive weight, high blood pressure, heart disease, diabetes and a family history of stroke. Other factors are unhealthy lifestyles and habits such as smoking, poor diet, and lack of exercise.

Strokes are caused by a blockage or lack of blood supply to specific areas of the brain, which can leave lasting neurological problems. These problems may include weakness, difficulty moving, and even paralysis.

A patient who has had a stroke must be evaluated and examined carefully to be certain the problem is disc or spinal nerve related. The DRS Protocol™ cannot improve any permanent damage caused by a stroke, but disc-related pain can be helped, and that will improve the patient's mobility. Stroke patients often experience a change in gait or function due to weakness in limbs on one side of the body.

These changes can cause the spine to twist into unnatural positions as the patient tries to compensate for the biomechanical deficiencies that cause pain. The pain, if determined to be from a disc problem, can be treated by the DRS Protocol™, and treatement will help improve function. The expectation for improvement is similar to that of any other patient.

Transplant Patients

Once very rare, there are now thousands of people who have had organ transplants. Most transplant recipients must stay on anti-rejection drugs for the remainder of their lives to ensure their bodies do not reject the transplanted organ. These drugs suppress the immune system. A patient with a transplant is treated as any other immune-suppressed patient. They are evaluated and monitored carefully.

When it is determined that the back or neck condition is appropriate for treatment with the DRS Protocol™, treatment is begun, and the patient's progress is followed closely. I have treated two heart transplant recipients and several kidney transplant recipients, all with excellent results.

It is important to be aware of all medications that the transplant patient is taking. I do not introduce any nutritional supplements without the advice of the transplant specialist. While transplant patients may require increased treatment time, it has been my experience that they respond very well.

Amputees

I have treated many amputees. Lower extremity amputations often affect the spine because the amputation naturally affects how the amputee bears weight. The gait and biomechanical function of an amputee is changed forever. Change of structure and function puts additional pressure on the spine and over time will cause degeneration of the spine and surrounding structures that are overstressed.

A patient of mine, Dave, had a dramatic story with a great outcome. Dave was involved in a terrible motorcycle accident. He eventually lost his leg just above the knee, and he was fitted with a prosthetic leg. As he was recovering and going through physical therapy to learn to use his new leg, he experienced significant pain. He was told that this was normal and he was experiencing phantom pain.

Phantom pain is a common occurrence in which the nerves send signals to the brain so that the brain perceives the amputated limb is still attached. The patient continues to feel pain. Nothing Dave tried successfully alleviated the pain.

Dave came for evaluation on the chance that I could alleviate any pain. His examination was difficult to perform. The normal orthopedic maneuvers used for evaluation had to be altered due to his missing leg.

Within the first week of treatment with the DRS Protocol™, Dave was amazed at how well his body had responded. He stated that 80% of the time, he did not feel any pain in his low back or leg. By the end of the course of treatment, his pain was completely gone. He was not experiencing phantom pain. Dave's real problems were related to his new prosthetic leg.

The problem was two-fold. First, he was walking on an unsteady and uneven foundation. The prosthetic leg was not an even length with his other leg, and therefore he was functioning with legs of different lengths. His orthopedic doctor corrected this part of the problem. The second problem was that as he learned to walk with his prosthetic leg, his natural gait was altered. This biomechanical change added to the problem.

Dave's story highlights the fact that there may be more than one answer when dealing with the human body. He, no doubt, originally had some phantom pain, as many amputees do. However, a large source of his pain was the result of a degenerative disc condition. Prior to his accident, Dave had a degenerative disc that I had successfully treated, and since his accident he had new symptoms. His major symptoms were resolved by treating with the DRS Protocol™. *Surgery not Included.*

Mental Degenerative Diseases

I frequently treat patients who are suffering from different degrees of Alzheimer's or dementia. It is estimated that five million people in the United States currently have Alzheimer's, which is considered the most common type of dementia. Alzheimer's destroys a person's brain cells, and it is slowly incapacitating. Over time, it is fatal and is currently the sixth leading cause of death in America. Dementia is a general term used to describe cognitive degeneration stemming from a variety of reasons. Many people with dementia have Alzheimer's, but not all.

Vascular dementia is caused by a narrowing of the blood vessels, thereby causing the blood supply to be cut off from the brain. The effect is similar to that of a stroke.

Both Alzheimer's and dementia are progressive neurological diseases of the brain that lead to impairment in memory, judgment, decision-making, speech, and orientation to surroundings. People with these diseases can exhibit strange behavior, and they can easily injure themselves or cause damage to their back and neck. Even those who are largely mentally incapacitated will still respond to treatment, and they certainly deserve to live free of pain.

Of course, with patients who have Alzheimer's or any form of dementia, I require that a family member who is in charge of healthcare decisions be present for any treatment decisions.

Parkinson's is another degenerative disease seen in patients generally over 50 years old. The disease may start with mild tremors in one hand; as the dopamine-producing cells in the brain degenerate, uncontrollable tremors occur in various parts of the body. Patients will have a change in gait, and their arms do not swing while walking, which causes them to lean forward and may even cause them to fall.

Part of the progression of Parkinson's is diminished reflexes. Therefore, if the patient is continually leaning forward or stooping over, this creates back and neck pain because the body has altered biomechanics. Patients with Parkinson's will also respond well to treatment for disc-related conditions.

Many symptoms of degenerative neurological diseases such as Parkinson's, Alzheimer's, dementia, and others will not directly respond to the DRS Protocol™. The DRS Protocol™ will alleviate pain in the back and neck related to disc conditions. It will not slow the progression of the neurological diseases.

Patients with other pre-existing health conditions will benefit from treatment with the DRS Protocol™ for the appropriate neck and back conditions. It only takes a short time to perform an evaluation that will determine if a patient is a candidate.

My mind always returns to my friend who assumed his father was not in good enough health to have treatment and his father did not believe in alternatives. His father opted for surgery instead and died during that surgery.

I cannot help but believe that had he decided on a nonsurgical treatment, he would have had many more good years with his family. Never assume someone is not a candidate for the DRS Protocol™ until a qualified evaluation has been performed.

Dr. Richard Busch III

CHAPTER 5
Other Treatments

CHAPTER 5
Other Treatments

Many patients, before coming to my office, have already undergone other types of treatment for back or neck pain. Often, treatment is considered effective even though only short-term relief is the expected outcome. Other treatments are not effective at all.

Long-term relief is statistically not the rule when dealing with the conventional treatment of herniated discs. I want to discuss some other treatment options that you may have tried or heard about, and either had a good experience or a disappointing one. I would like to encourage you that no matter what your previous experiences were with any other treatments; you can still have a good experience with spinal decompression when the DRS Protocol™ is used.

Much non-emergency medical information is obtained from people we know other than a doctor: the neighbor, the friend at church, or the person at work. That is the method we use to find the best sales, the favorite restaurants, and the movies that are worth seeing. People often share medical advice. This may lead to misinformation about medical conditions and which treatment is right for you.

This word-of-mouth information is also how we can find doctors that are liked. However, it does not excuse us from becoming knowledgeable enough to ask competent questions and find the right care. Just because your Aunt Tilly suffered back pain for years, does not mean that you have to suffer!

Late-Night Remedies

Who has not occasionally stayed up late at night watching infomercials and been tempted to order a special pillow or a lightweight vacuum, just in case it is as great as advertised? Back or neck pain sufferers often have insomnia, and they frequently find themselves channel surfing on late-night television. When patients are dissatisfied with medical options, or their personal treatment outcomes, or perhaps they have a deep-seated fear of doctors, they may start buying products and programs that seem to offer hope to solve their chronic problem. In addition, many patients feel lonely and abandoned because of their problems. Watching an infomercial may feel like joining a family. The offers may include vitamin programs, exercise regimens, massage chairs, gravity boots, and various inversion tables or mechanical devices that purport to relieve back pain. Sometimes, patients do experience temporary relief, but it rarely lasts long, and there is a very real potential to aggravate the problem rather than cure it.

The majority of the time the products do not do a thing to improve the situation. The patient is still in pain, albeit a little lighter in the wallet. It is important to note, there is a reason infomercials state that *individual results may vary*: they vary widely!

Drugs

Patients will often try to alleviate a pain problem themselves by taking larger doses of over-the-counter (OTC) medications. This includes NSAIDs (nonsteroidal anti-inflammatory drugs) such as aspirin and ibuprofen.

Once a patient decides to see a doctor, the first step in alleviating back pain for most medical professionals may be to recommend continuing the OTC pain relievers like Tylenol. Patients must be very careful not take too much because even though products are OTC, they can cause serious side effects. OTC topical pain relievers like analgesic patches or topical ointments may be recommended. If the OTC products do not help, doctors then may prescribe muscle relaxants and/or anti-inflammatories. However, they also have potential side effects. Anti-inflammatories may include steroids.

Steroids are useful in the short term, and I occasionally will recommend that patients secure treatment from their general practitioner to get the inflammation under control. Nevertheless, steroids are meant for short-term use and do have side effects.

One of the more noticeable side effects is weight gain and water retention. Patients on long-term use of steroids tend to have round "baby" faces and put on extra pounds. Prolonged use of steroids can cause soft tissue damage such as accelerated degeneration of the cartilage, bone weakness, and osteoporotic changes—which is exactly what we need to avoid—so the use of steroids should be brief and infrequent.

A doctor may prescribe oral steroids such as cortisone or steroid injections. The body produces cortisol, and cortisone is a synthetic reproduction of this natural substance. An injection of these medications maximizes the anti-inflammatory effect more quickly than taking oral medications. The objective of this course of action is to allow the inflammation to decrease and to allow the patient's body time to heal.

Drugs are never a long-term solution. The body's ability to adapt means that many drugs are less effective over time. The body compensates and begins to create the inflammation again, which is why an increased number of drugs or more powerful drugs must be prescribed. Eventually, there is a limit to this course of treatment.

Family doctors are very reluctant to prescribe pain medications because the US Centers for Disease Control Preventions have issued new guidelines, as there have been over 72,000 deaths in 2017 reported due to pain medications.[1] The guidelines state that primary care doctors must closely monitor their patients' opioid prescription use and to limit prescriptions in the effort to stop drug abuse, overdosing and creating drug dependency.

Even though primary physicians can prescribe pain medications, it is most likely they will refer the back pain patient to a surgeon or a pain specialist.

CBD (Cannabidiol)

It is an understatement to say that CBD has had an explosion in alternative medicine, it is still relatively new in the literature but you can hardly turn on a news program or read a magazine without seeing some article or story on its benefits, especially for pain. It is also constantly on social media.

CBD is a natural substance derived from the cannabis plant which also contains hemp and marijuana. However, CBD contains little to no THC, the psychoactive ingredient in marijuana that makes people feel 'high'. The hype around CBD is due to it showing promise for pain relief with few to any of the side effects of opioids or other drugs. The danger, however, is that it is being touted as curing everything from anxiety to cancer and has been so overhyped that it is quickly becoming the modern-day version of snake oil.

Studies have already shown that certain forms of CBD does have a positive effect on certain types of epilepsy and has also been shown to relieve anxiety and help patients sleep. There is also a study that has shown it may have a therapeutic effect on inflammation and pain.

So what's the problem? The main issue here is that there haven't been many good, large studies of the effects of CBD for a variety of specific uses such as acute or chronic back pain. That may not sound like a big deal, but it is. Large, well conducted scientific studies are how we learn what side effects a substance may have, what the possible drug interactions may be and what dose to use for a specific outcome.

Since very little of that type of study has been done specifically for acute and chronic pain relief, and the manufacture of CBD is largely unregulated (as of this writing), people are just guessing what conditions it might work for and what dose might be helpful.

It is also difficult to know which manufacturer is producing a good quality product so strength and potency vary wildly.

It is important to understand that every supplement, vitamin or drug has a therapeutic dosage and use. This means that through study we know that 160mg of aspirin might give slight relief for pain and produce few, if any, side effects. But 5000mg of aspirin can be disastrous long-term and produce a number of side effects. Even compounds we think are good for us, like vitamins, can be toxic at the wrong dosage or produce side effects when combined with other substances.

I'm not saying CBD should not be used for pain, I'm sure it does, and will, have some good applications, but we must use caution before assuming it will work for every patient or every circumstance. We need more empirical data before we start experimenting on people who are so desperate for pain relief they will do almost anything.

This brings up the 'more is better' conundrum. It is human nature to assume that if one pill of something is good, more is better. We see it constantly in patients who overuse supplements, OTC drugs and harsh dietary regimes. But it is, in fact, not true. More is not better, oftentimes it's just more and either has a detrimental effect or no additional effect at all except to cost the patient money.

This is why it is so important to discuss everything you are taking with your doctor in order to come up with a comprehensive health plan. Everything affects everything and while CBD may be a good source of pain relief for many patients, it needs to be monitored and patients must be wary of claims that are too good to be true.

In summary, we have been seeing a great response for patients with chronic and acute pain in using CBD. I do think it can be an important adjunct for the patient in chronic pain and may help lower the need for harsher drugs. I do also think that it is being over sold and emphasized as the cure-all for everything which is simply not true. It will have its uses, but it won't fix the underlying issues causing the pain.

Injections

Injections may be performed for back or neck pain. If there is any relief, it is often short-lived. Sometimes the injections provide no relief, depending on many factors and a patient's history. There are varying types of injections, and the most prevalent types include epidural, selective nerve root block (SNRB), facet joint block, facet rhizotomy (an ablation), and sacroiliac joint block.

Epidurals are routinely used as an attempt to relieve back or neck pain temporarily. The medication, which usually contains an anti-inflammatory to reduce inflammation, is injected directly into the epidural space. This space surrounds the spinal cord and contains lymphatics, nerves, and spinal fluid.

The SNRB is a diagnostic procedure performed to determine which spinal nerve root is the origin of pain in an attempt to gain therapeutic pain relief from inflammation at that nerve root. If there is a reduction of pain from an SNRB, then a radio frequency nerve ablation will be performed to destroy the nerve that is diagnosed as causing the pain. The SNRB is also performed for the facet joint and sacroiliac joint, but again the results, if any, are short-term and therapeutic.

Each progressive injection may be less effective. The effectiveness will vary with each patient. Initially, the injections may be beneficial in blocking the pain or decreasing the inflammation, but in the end, these do not help a patient heal. It buys time, but it is not a cure for the condition. Patients who have had these injections often have said it acted much like a band-aid. They had pain relief for a week or a few months, at best. Inevitably, their pain returned.

One concern about the continued use of pain medications and anti-inflammatories is these simply mask the pain. Without pain, the patient may continue to perform certain activities or movements that could cause damage to the injured area. The injured area could experience significant degeneration from repetitive injury and the continued use of steroids. According to one school of thought, if you continue to exercise a joint that is not moving correctly, this may accelerate degeneration of the injured joint by up to thirty percent.

A more aggressive treatment is facet rhizotomy injection. If a patient had some temporary relief with a series of facet block injections, then the procedure, facet rhizotomy injection, may be performed in which a needle with a probe is inserted near the nerves around the facet joint of the spine. The probe, heated by radio waves, is applied to the sensory nerve related to the facet joint. In theory, this kills the nerve to the joint capsule, which stops pain signals from going to the brain. This technique is also called a nerve ablation, and it burns and destroys the nerves. The ablation may cause increased pain later.

Physical Therapy

Physical therapy (PT) is the use of designed exercises and equipment to rehabilitate an injury. Physical therapy is often used in conjunction with medication and injections for neck and back pain. The goal is to help extend a patient's range of motion, strengthen muscles, decrease pain, and resume normal activities.

Physical therapists educate and instruct the patient on how to work, lift, and move without further injury. Again, many patients who have severe disc conditions end up frustrated because physical therapy rarely changes function enough to correct a problem for the long term, or to avoid surgery.

When an exercise program is prescribed, usually one of two things happens: either pain increases or relief is short-lived. Severe pain can limit the ability to bend, stretch, and move. While physical therapy is valuable for treating a serious traumatic injury or a surgical procedure that has damaged muscles that need to be strengthened, it is my opinion that physical therapy is not as effective for disc-related conditions. In fact, it may cause an exacerbation of the condition. Many of my patients, who were referred to physical therapy, complained that after physical therapy, their symptoms were worse.

Complementary and Alternative Medical Therapies

Complementary and alternative medicine (CAM) is a group of diverse medical and healthcare systems, practices, and products. CAM therapies, according to Mayo Clinic, have never been more popular. The popularity of CAM therapies is on the rise as at least 40% of adults in the United States use some type of these therapies according to the National Center of Complementary Medicine. The following are only a few of the common CAM therapies.

Acupuncture, while licensed in certain states in the United States, has been one of the principal forms of treatment in traditional Chinese medicine, and it has been practiced for more than 5,000 years. The perspective from which an acupuncturist views health and sickness is the concept of balanced energy.

Acupuncture treatment consists of placing very thin stainless steel needles into the skin of the patient at specific locations— meridian points—that correspond to certain parts of the body associated with energy channels. The goal of acupuncture is to balance the body's chi, or life force. This treatment has been used for thousands of years for a range of problems, including pain. While it can help on a temporary basis, it is not a long-term treatment for pain associated with spinal disc conditions.

Dietary supplements are considered a CAM therapy and can be as basic as the vitamins I offer most of my patients as part of their treatment protocol: Vitamins such as vitamin B's, vitamin C, and calcium with magnesium. Each plays an important part in aiding the body to maximize healing. If needed, enzyme therapy can be an additional part of a patient's treatment. Enzyme therapy helps the body's ability to break down nutrients.

Another part of CAM supplementation therapy can be herbal remedies like ginseng, echinacea, and ginkgo among many others. Some supplementation can be very simple, and others are complex and even compounded. It is important to take high-quality supplementation as not all products are created equal, and many are manufactured with synthetic chemicals.

Homeopathy, a CAM therapy, is the belief that the body can heal itself based on the philosophy of "like cures like," utilizing almost less than detectable levels of natural products in liquids, usually alcohol or water. Homeopathic remedies are very popular in Europe and are viewed as effective for conditions like hay fever and allergies in the United States.

Chiropractic is the practice of diagnosing and treating of neuromusculoskeletal disorders of the spine and their effects on the nervous system. Chiropractic care involves treating with manipulation of the spine, joints and extremities, and soft tissue. Chiropractic care can offer multiple therapies along with manipulation and is considered to be the best choice for conservative treatment of back and neck pain based on studies showing overall positive outcomes and little to no recovery time.

Mind and body practices are excellent for strengthening the relationship between the mind and body. A popular example is yoga, as it stresses posture, breathing, meditation, and relaxation. Even though yoga is physical, it is considered a spiritual practice, as is prayer.

Guided imagery, also CAM therapy, is the concept of the mind and body being interconnected and influencing each other. Clinical studies have shown that imagery, or visualization, can affect the physiological responses of the heart, respiratory system, immune functions, cellular growth, pain, relaxation, and sleep. With the DRS Protocol™, all of my patients receive instruction in visualization or guided imagery.

Homeopathic and guided imagery are often beyond what is offered in a traditional clinical setting. Medical doctors offer a wide array of surgical and diagnostic procedures, but many set aside natural healing ideas.

Traditional Surgical Interventions and Diagnostic Procedures

There are two different categories of surgical procedures: diagnostic and intervention. Diagnostics include procedures such as a discogram, which is a diagnostic procedure performed before a surgery. It is performed to determine definitively which disc is causing the pain and if a fusion is required.

During a discogram, the doctor slides a needle through the body (through the abdomen if the problem is in the lumbar region) while the patient is awake, though the patient is usually sedated. A sterile saline solution with a radiologic dye is injected into the disc, and the pain response is recorded (a positive finding is the re-creation of the actual pain previously reported by the patient). Guided fluoroscopic images (moving X-rays) are made, and the damaged disc is shown on film during the discogram.

Discograms are extremely painful, and someone needs to drive the patient home afterward. It may cause nerve damage in the disc, and it accelerates degeneration of the disc. I believe that a thorough examination and a medical history, along with an X-ray or MRI, will give the same information, in most cases.

A myelogram is an X-ray study in which dye is injected into the cerebrospinal fluid, and then the patient is X-rayed to see if there is pressure on the nerves of the spinal cord coming from the disc. This study is important because, during the study, the patient's head and torso are raised to a 45º angle. The body, at this angle, puts pressure on the disc, and this shows how the disc might appear in a weight-bearing situation. One very serious side effect of the procedure can be arachnoiditis. This is inflammation of the tissue covering the spinal cord, causing severe, long-term pain and neurological problems. There is no cure for arachnoiditis.

Should the patient opt for surgical intervention, there are also different methods for surgery, depending on the surgeon's specialization and the patient's condition. A discectomy is a procedure to shave off the bulging portion of the disc.

Unfortunately, the disc often becomes weaker in the area where the procedure was performed and much more vulnerable to injury. Some doctors perform a discectomy with an arthroscopic laser. The laser will burn off the bulging portion of the disc, while other doctors surgically cut away a portion of the disc.

As with any surgical procedure, there is always the dilemma of the formation of scar tissue (epidural fibrosis), and it is very common. Some doctors inform their patients that scar tissue can form and surgery for its removal may be required.

Surgery for the removal of scar tissue may need to be repeated. If the removal of scar tissue does not improve their pain, then patients must turn to pain management techniques to help with it.

Another spinal surgery is fusion, and there are different surgical procedures that may be used for spinal fusion. They differ in the surgical approach – through the front, back, or side of the body - and the instrumentation used. All have advantages and disadvantages.

A current surgical procedure used for some fusions is minimally invasive surgery (MIS), meaning the surgery is performed using a smaller incision opening. The goal is to cause the smallest amount of trauma and damage to tissue and muscle from the actual surgery. It is a very complex surgery and requires the highest technical expertise. Each surgery, open and minimally invasive, is not without important advantages and disadvantages

The purpose of a fusion surgery is to stop the movement of the vertebrae, immobilize that injured part of the spine, and then allow new grafted bone to grow and stabilize the fused area into a static position. The stabilization can be accomplished by instrumented fusion, which is done by inserting titanium rods on either side of the spine and locking them in place with screws, or by implanting titanium cages. Each has a different surgical approach.

Usually, cages in the lumbar spine are implanted through an incision in the front of the body, and rods are implanted through the back. Each implantation has its risks. Cages have a higher risk of nonfusion and of causing bleeding.

For males, there is a chance of retrograde ejaculation because of potential damage to nerves. Each type of fusion can be partnered with bone implants: cadaver bone (harvested from a cadaver), synthetic bone, or bone from the patient's own donation. However, donations can have a relatively high risk of complication such as chronic pain after surgery, infection, and pelvic fractures, all associated with the area of the bone harvest.

It can take months—up to 12 months in some cases—for the surgery to heal and stabilize. The problem with spinal fusions is they do not reliably provide long-term positive outcomes, and the patient may be free of pain for only two to three years, if ever.

When a fusion is completed, the vertebrae directly above and below the fusion tend to experience accelerated degeneration and are likely to cause a future problem, requiring additional surgery to fuse the adjacent vertebral levels. A successful fusion is judged on whether it eliminates movement at the fused level— not whether the surgery has reduced pain.

A recent study about fusions was presented that unveiled a surprising answer to the following question, "Have specialists [surgeons] been exaggerating the degree to which spinal fusion for low back pain is a successful operation?" And the answer was an undisputed "yes" as reported in *The Back Letter,* Vol 33 No 5, 2018.[2] This study reviewed fusion patients and their outcomes over time. The result was about 38% improvement in pain. Surgeons from other specialties, such and hip and knee replacement, would say that 38% is a very low number, and that this type of surgery [fusion] is a failure.

There are many studies such as "Lumbar Fusion Compared with Conservative Treatment in Patients with Chronic Back Pain" published in the *International Journal of Rehabilitation Research*, that conclude there is not sufficient evidence to show that lumbar fusions provide greater improvement for back pain than alternative conservative treatment.[3]

Conservative treatment would include chiropractic care, back education, cognitive behavioral therapy, physical therapy, exercise, weight reduction, and other alternative therapies.

The DRS Protocol™ can improve pain from the disc problem of the level above and below the fused portion of the spine, but nothing can be done to change the fused area. Despite the uncertainty of fusions, lumbar fusion surgeries are still rapidly increasing.

The United States has the highest rates of fusions in the world, and about fifty percent are being performed on patients with diagnoses that experts and insurance companies say should not be treated with fusions.

Another surgical procedure for degenerative disc disease is disc replacement, and there are several types of replacement implants. Simply explained, this surgery involves removing the "target disc" – the one diagnosed as causing pain - and replacing it with an artificial implant made of metal or polymer. These procedures are performed for degenerative disc disease primarily of the lumbar and cervical spine.

Artificial Disc Replacement surgery (ADR) was approved for the public in 2004. The hope was that this emerging technology would revolutionize spine surgery and have better outcomes than fusions (success rate of about 38%) as a cure to treat certain spine conditions such as degenerative disc disease.

The goal of the ADR is to relieve pain and imitate the motion of a normal spine, unlike fusions that limit spine mobility. At this time, ADR surgery has a success rate of about 40%

Many surgeons are reluctant to perform disc replacements because there are few long-term studies and it is early in clinical experience, (many candidates are young people). The procedure is considered an emerging technology with success rates about the same as fusions.

As Michael Fehling MD, a surgeon who regularly performs disc replacements said, "But the patient must be wary because not all patients can expect to be "normal", and "Patients should also be aware that the long-term outcomes of artificial discs are still not well-known and that revision surgery may be required down the road."[4]

One frequent question from many of my patients is, "Can't a bad disc just be replaced with a good one?" Disc replacement is still in the early phases, and there is no real understanding of how they will work in the long-term. It has been shown that adjacent discs will have accelerated degeneration and additional surgeries will be required.

In my opinion, this is a whole new treatment spectrum with great risks. If revision surgery is required, the procedure can be life-threatening. I believe patients should consider alternative therapies, if at all possible. Once disc replacement surgery has been performed, patients cannot be treated with the DRS Protocol™.

Decompressive laminectomy is a surgical procedure that removes a piece of the bony arch, or lamina, on the dorsal surface of a vertebra. It is much like lifting the top of a tunnel. A portion of the vertebra is lifted off exposing the spinal cord to relieve pressure on the spinal cord and nerves.

With age, discs begin to degenerate, and the vertebrae in the spine become much closer to each other. This can result in bone spurs and ligamentum flavum in hypertrophy (a condition where the spinal canal narrows, causing spinal stenosis and pressure on the nerves). These changes can cause the spinal canal and the foramina, the small opening in the vertebra, to narrow, which may pinch the spinal nerves. Different studies report different success rates, and even surgeons' success rates will differ. Laminectomies were performed more routinely in the past. However, they are still being done.

Patients who have had any of these previous surgeries and are still in pain can have good results with the DRS Protocol™, with the exception of those who have had a disc replacement.

Patients who have disc surgery have a variance in outcomes, with most falling into the areas described below. Outcomes may also be influenced by age, diagnosis, and other health conditions.

1. Little or no improvement: According to recent studies, approximately 40% of patients who undergo spinal surgery have little or no improvement. Although pain might change from a sharp pain to a dull aching pain, surgery really provides no relief. It is common for radiating pain in the leg or arm to be resolved by surgery, but a patient may continue to experience a considerable amount of back or neck pain.

2. Moderate improvement: Another 20% saw moderate improvement while 40% had improvement one-year post surgery. Of course, there are patients who will have excellent results, though it is not very common. Even those who initially show improvement will statistically be more likely to experience problems within a few years. Although it is very difficult to pin down the exact figures, it is reported by many studies that conservatively 20% to 40% and even up to 74% of patients have not experienced success in alleviating pain after surgical intervention for back pain. Perhaps the problem is due to underreporting of ongoing problems suffered by patients and the overuse of surgery as a cure for pain. This means that surgery is routinely recommended for patients who have other health conditions that will interfere with their ability to have a successful outcome, and the results can be very disappointing.

3. Worse pain following surgery: This is very common, as often the surgery injures other tissue and causes scar tissue to form that creates more pain. Additional causes can be inaccurate diagnoses, misdiagnoses, and poor choice of surgical candidates.

4. Permanent damage, numbness, muscle weakness, or muscle atrophy: Any of these outcomes is possible. When the body is cut open, damage can be done to vital structures within the spine, which can cause permanent damage and disability.

5. All other risks inherent in surgery: Other risks include infection and even death. Even when patients feel their surgery has had a good outcome because they initially feel better, they do not realize how much weaker their spine is after surgery.

Jack's story is a sad, yet strong, example of this point. He had previously had a discectomy, the surgical removal of part or all of a vertebral disc that has herniated. Jack was pleased with the outcome at that point. Two weeks later, as he was returning for his post-surgical follow-up examination, he had an unfortunate experience. He was on the elevator, and it stopped just a few inches above the floor level. Jack did not notice. As he walked off the elevator, he stepped down hard and jolted his back. He reherniated the same disc, right there in the medical building.

Jack came to me for treatment with the DRS Protocol™ because he absolutely was not going through surgery again. Surgery is a traumatic procedure for any part of the body, let alone the spine. He felt that if his spine was that weak after the first surgery, then he did not want to go through it again and have the risk of continuing pain.

Even if a patient has failed back or neck surgery and is experiencing post-surgery pain, he or she can begin DRS Protocol™. The waiting period is only four to six weeks. However, if a patient has had a spinal fusion, where bone and instrumentation were implanted, the required wait is at least six to eight months. This allows time for the bone and surrounding tissue to heal completely and become as stable as possible.

It is important to remember that the fused level of the patient's spine will not be able to be treated. However, the adjacent levels above and below the fusion can be treated with the DRS Protocol™. Patient welfare and a good outcome are paramount to me.

Spinal Cord Stimulators (SCS)

Patients still experiencing post-surgical pain because of failed surgery for a disc condition will often have to move into a pain management program. Ultimately, pain pumps and spinal cord stimulators (SCS) are prescribed in an attempt to maintain patients' pain at a livable level. The pain pump is a small device implanted under the skin and intermittently injects medication directly into the spinal cord.

There are inconveniences and risks involved with a pain pump. Pain medications need to be pre-ordered and refilled through a specialist. Side effects from the medications are common and must be monitored to adjust the dose. Batteries and regular maintenance are required. The patient has a process to go through for approval, and healing time is about six weeks. Results vary greatly depending on the cause and severity of the patient's pain.

Spinal cord stimulators are another alternative to help control of pain from failed back surgeries, chronic pain, and nerve damage. A small wire or lead, which connects to a power source, is implanted surgically in the spinal cord. Electrical signals are transmitted through the lead to the spinal cord or to specific nerves to block pain signals from reaching the brain.

Some stimulators use a remote control to turn the current off or on and to adjust intensity. There are two types: one is an implanted unit that uses a pulse generator and a non-rechargeable battery that is replaced over time. The second system employs radio frequencies, and it uses a transmitter with an antenna, which is much like a cell phone and a receiver that is implanted in the body. The patient has to have had a successful trial period with the spinal cord stimulator before a permanent stimulator is implanted.

Pain is the body's means of communicating there is a problem. Spinal cord stimulation interferes with nerve transmission of pain. It does not address the underlying problem. Possible risks of spinal cord stimulators include hardware failure, lead migration or breakage, and scar tissue (fibrosis) formation around the electrode. These may cause nerve damage, which can include progressive quadriparesis (gradually weakening of the arms and legs). There can be an actual increase in pain and the reduction of the effectiveness of the stimulator.

Additional surgery may be required to replace an SCS if there are complications. Researchers have found that nearly 10 percent of patients who have had an SCS have suffered some degree of damage to the spinal cord or the spinal nerve root.

Another problem is the patient may have pain that gradually moves beyond the reach of the nerve stimulator, rendering it useless. In addition, the patient's body may compensate, and the stimulator could become less effective.

Paralysis can occur with an SCS, however at relatively low rate. SCS's can be the cause of other complications such as scarring from battery pack, electrodes that can't be removed and the inability to have MRI's performed on the patient again. Many patients don't recall being informed about not ever being able to have another MRI – even if the patient has cancer or a stroke.

The implantation of a foreign object in the body has the risk of causing infection in the spine. Spinal cord stimulators or pain pumps can cause the leakage of spinal fluid and disabling headaches. The increased stimulation from SCS's may also cause bladder problems.

Treatment success with SCS's is influenced by the cause of pain, if there has been a previous back surgery, and the amount of time that has passed since the surgery. The longer the time since a first surgery, the less likely the SCS will overpower the pain signals that have developed. Often, when a SCS stops working, it is just left inside the patient. It is not removed or replaced.

When I consult with a patient who has a working SCS, I do not treat the area where the stimulator is implanted. If the patient's implant is not working, then it is preferable to have the stimulator removed before beginning treatment with the DRS Protocol™. There are many reasons to be cautious with SCS's. The primary reason is the leads can be pulled out of place with spinal decompression treatment or chiropractic manipulation.

Chiropractic Care and Spinal Decompression

Chiropractic, by definition of the American Chiropractic Association, is a healthcare profession that focuses on disorders of the musculoskeletal system, and the nervous system and the effects these disorders have on overall health. Chiropractic care is used most often to treat back pain, neck pain, headaches, and pain in the joints of the arms or legs.

Chiropractors perform spinal manipulations or spinal adjustments in order to restore function of the nervous system and the spine, which alleviates the pressure on the nerves, muscle tightness, pain, and allows the tissue to heal.

Spinal manipulation does not hurt. However, occasionally a patient may experience very mild soreness, perhaps for some it is like the feeling after working out for the first time. Doctors of Chiropractic do not prescribe drugs or perform surgery.

Traditional chiropractic care is very effective in conservative care and management of back and neck pain and disc-related conditions. However, there is a level of severity of a disc condition that surpasses the effectiveness of treatment with standard chiropractic care.

The DRS Protocol™ is comprised of spinal decompression, multiple therapies, specific chiropractic manipulation, nutrition, and exercise to provide an encompassing treatment and management protocol for chronic and severe disc conditions.

A patient with a disc condition may have previously responded to chiropractic care, but as the condition progressively worsens there may be a limit to what chiropractic treatment can do for continued improvement. For these patients, I treat with the DRS Protocol™, and improvement is seen quickly. Naturally, each patient progresses according to the diagnosis, lifestyle, habits, and other health factors.

Both chiropractic and spinal decompression are gentle and noninvasive and are intended to restore normal function to the body. They work well together and allow the body to heal naturally. Spinal decompression, which is safe and pain-free, employs a computerized distractive force over a logarithmic curve. This process can override the body's natural defense mechanism of tightening the muscles in response to external pulling.

This logarithmic curve allows the application of specific amounts of force to be applied to the spine directly at the level of the disc injury, either of the lumbar or cervical spine. The angle of that specific force targets the disc level to be treated.

Spinal decompression employs a computerized program with patient-specific parameters, angles, and weight-of-pull that is customized and can be retained in the software for each individual. Most importantly, spinal decompression uses the application of ramping, which slowly introduces axial force to the spine.

This creates a wider spacing of the vertebral discs, which in turn, creates a negative internal disc pressure (decompression). The bulging material from the disc will naturally retract back into the disc and off of the spinal cord and nerves.

The DRS Protocol™ is a successful system of treatment elements: spinal decompression, chiropractic care, and other therapies and elements that facilitate healing. I am offering my patients a choice that is a successful alternative to surgery.

The protocol meets a full range of patient needs and helps to facilitate healing. Patients can expect outcomes in the following categories:

1.High percentage of improvement or dramatic improvement: There is frequently 100% improvement, which means the patient is back to a normal life and pain-free.

2.Large percentage improvement with decreased pain and less muscle spasm: Patients may have more strength but will not be completely back to the way they were pre-injury. However, patients have achieved substantial improvement and will return to a normal, full lifestyle. The patient who has had long-standing degenerative disc disease pain may now only notice pain when the area is aggravated by a specific activity.

3.Patient responds well to treatment and has had pain for so long that the improvement is life-altering, although the condition is not totally resolved: The patient who has had long-standing degenerative pain may still be limited in certain activities but will be largely improved.

4.Patient has improvement in some areas, but not all: There is improvement in some areas of complaint, but the results are not dramatic. This category represents a small percentage of all patients.

Nowhere in the list does death or spinal cord damage appear, nor do any other inherent risks of surgery appear or apply to the DRS Protocol™. This particular point alone makes a particularly convincing reason to research conservative, noninvasive care.

Dr. Richard Busch III

CHAPTER 6
Beyond Back and Neck Pain

CHAPTER 6
Beyond Back and Neck Pain

I have told my patients through the years, "We treat pain." Since 1996, this primarily meant back and neck pain. However, over time while treating patients with spinal conditions like degenerative disc disease and herniated discs with the DRS Protocol™, many of these patients also had symptoms characteristic of peripheral neuropathy as well.

Some of their symptoms were of pain, but they also had numbness and tingling in the arms and hands or legs and feet, feeling cold, loss of feeling, and loss of balance among other problems.

Some of these patients had been diagnosed with diabetic neuropathy. With treatment, their back and neck problems were corrected, and many found their neuropathy symptoms resolved because their neuropathy symptoms resulted from mechanical causes and not diabetes or other causes.

Through my years of practice, there has been a definite increase in the number of patients suffering from peripheral neuropathy. There can be over a hundred causes; however, peripheral neuropathy is commonly associated with chemotherapy and diabetes.

The increase is understandable, as diabetes is escalating at an alarming rate, and close to 50 percent of people with diabetes are afflicted with peripheral neuropathy. The sharp rise of type 2 diabetes can be attributed to lifestyle factors, weight, food additives, and cholesterol medications (statins).

Seeing the negative impact neuropathy has had on many patients' lives, I was highly motivated to find treatment to help patients with their peripheral neuropathy symptoms without exposing them to harmful medications and other painful testing. Soon, I began developing the Busch Neuropathy Protocol™, which has treatment guidelines with multiple treatment elements including whole body vibration, laser therapy, infrared and photomodulation therapy for tissue repair, specific nutritional supplementation, and chiropractic therapies and techniques.

Treatment with the Busch Neuropathy Protocol™ has been a pivotal treatment experience for my patients. Many who had already been deeply disappointed and were quietly suffering. This treatment protocol has been their answer!

A simple definition of neuropathy is death or damage of a nerve, and peripheral neuropathy develops from disorders or injuries to the peripheral nerves. These are nerves in our body, but outside of the nerves in the brain and spinal cord – (our central nervous system). The peripheral nervous system carries messages from our brains and spinal cords to every part of the body and then transports sensory messages back again.

These messages are sensory impulses sent back to the brain that let you feel, for example, hot or cold. These protective sensations let you know if you step on something sharp or stub your toes. They are also vital in communicating motor messages that determine where your feet are placed and how you move. Balance, walking and general movement can be affected both in large and small ways if these nerves are damaged.

Again, many symptoms may appear such as numbness or tingling in the hands and feet, shooting pain, feelings of cold or sensitivity to heat, and loss of balance. The pain and symptoms can become so intense that they can affect a person's ability to move around or sleep, and this markedly diminishes the quality of life.

Also, the Loss of Protective Sensations, (LOPS), is very dangerous because by not being able to feel painful sensations – a burn, a cut, a sore – an injury can easily occur. This can lead to greater damage and infection and can even cause the loss of a foot or leg to amputation.

Nerves control every function in our bodies, and these include internal organs and gland function. Because neuropathy can affect the organ and gland nerves, patients' symptoms may be mistaken for other diseases. The symptoms may include poor digestion, bloating or constipation, sweating, sexual impotence, and urination problems.

These similar symptoms can lead to a misdiagnosis, and neuropathy often simply goes undiagnosed. While the symptoms are treated, the underlying condition of neuropathy continues to worsen.

Since the symptoms of peripheral neuropathy usually develop over time and can come and go, many people just adapt to the increasing level of discomfort before they ever seek treatment. They frequently think it is just part of getting older to have pain and discomfort, so they let it go – until their problems become unbearable and prevent ordinary daily activities.

While, yes, some aches and pains come with advancing age, intense pain or symptoms that limit your life can be indicators of a much more serious condition and should be addressed as soon as possible. Diagnosing neuropathy early offers the best opportunity for controlling the problems of neuropathy, and there are treatment options for the pain and symptoms of neuropathy other than drugs.

Causes of Peripheral Neuropathy

Many patients diagnosed with peripheral neuropathy do not understand anything about their problem, as a clear explanation may have never been offered to the patient. I have found that helping patients make sense of their condition contributes to the best understanding of why they have the related problems.

This has helped them to overcome their fears, better manage their symptoms and certainly become more engaged with their care. All of which can result in even better treatment outcomes.

Often, as we do a comprehensive medical examination and thorough history of a patient, we will learn useful information that will help in the patient's treatment. Diabetes, medications for chemotherapy and cholesterol (statins), alcohol use, and even heredity are very common causes of neuropathy. Because the Busch Chiropractic Pain Center specializes in treating neuropathy symptoms with the Busch Neuropathy Protocol™ we are very familiar with symptoms of peripheral neuropathy and have a great deal of success in treating the neuropathy patient.

There are many causes of peripheral neuropathy, but we are going to focus on the types produced by disease processes or trauma, as they are by far the most prevalent.

Mechanical Neuropathy due to Physical Injury, Nerve Impingement or Trauma

Mechanical neuropathy comes from causes that we have treated for years with the DRS Protocol™. Many patients who have back and neck conditions of herniated and degenerative discs, spinal stenosis, and failed back surgery have neuropathy symptoms of pain, burning, tightness, numbness and tingling in the hands and arms or legs and feet.

These back and neck conditions are causing neuropathy symptoms because they are placing pressure on nerves as they leave the spine, and the nerves are being compressed.

Other causes of mechanical neuropathy are injuries from a sudden trauma or accident which can damage nerves either short-term or long-term and cause peripheral neuropathy. The damage could be resulting from auto accidents, sports injuries, surgeries or anything that causes the nerves to be pinched, stretched, crushed, severed or damaged in any way. Even something relatively minor like a dislocated joint can induce neuropathy.

Something we commonly see in patients is repetitive stress injuries. These stress injuries include carpal tunnel syndrome (CTS) with nerve entrapment in the wrist and ulnar neuropathy which is nerve entrapment usually at the elbow. Even though many don't think of CTS as a neuropathy, technically it is a neuropathy due to damage to the nerve.

Repetitive stress injuries are cumulative types of injuries that happen over an extended period of performing certain repeated movements. Moving joints in a recurrent pattern can cause ligaments and muscles to become inflamed and put pressure on surrounding nerves causing numbness, burning, pins and needles, weakness and pain. Repetitive stress injuries can be created by anything that incurs stress and strain on the forearm or wrist. The inflammation causes pressure on the nerve. Examples of job requirements that can produce repetitive stress injuries are working with power tools, cashiering and manufacturing work. Other factors that may contribute to CTS are rheumatoid arthritis and wrist fractures. They can put pressure on the median nerve in the wrist, and chronic diabetes can also cause damage to the median nerve.

Diseases and Disease Processes (Metabolic)

Neuropathy can also be triggered by various diseases or processes that cause disorders in the body. The leading cause of neuropathy in the US is diabetes. The following chapter is dedicated specifically to diabetic neuropathy because we are seeing a high percentage of patients who suffer from neuropathy related to their diabetes.

Other metabolic diseases that can cause neuropathies include anything that can cause hormonal imbalances such as underproduction of hormones produced by the thyroid gland or hypothyroidism (underactive thyroid). The imbalances can slow metabolism causing fluid retention and swollen tissues. This swelling presses on nerves and can cause pain. Some liver diseases will cause chemical imbalances that damage nerves, as well, leading to an onset of neuropathy.

Lupus, rheumatoid arthritis, and Guillain-Barre syndrome are just a few of the autoimmune diseases that are connected to peripheral neuropathy. An autoimmune disease is when the body attacks its own normal cells by mistake and can lead to nerve damage. Since many of these diseases go through periods of remission and relapse, they are considered chronic and will continue to damage tissue and nerves over time making pain and symptoms worse.

There are millions of people in the US with kidney disease, and few realize how this type of disease can cause long-term neuropathy symptoms. Nerves are very sensitive to toxins of most any nature, even toxins produced by your body. If kidney function is impaired, then waste or toxins will build up in the blood and cause damage to many types of cells including nerves. A majority of people who require dialysis due to kidney failure will experience some level of neuropathy.

Cancer can cause peripheral neuropathy. We already discussed some about chemotherapy being a cause, but cancer itself can also be the cause. Cancers can put pressure on surrounding nerve tissues and can also develop in the nerve cells themselves. Of course, toxicity from treatments for cancer, including chemotherapy, is well known for producing peripheral neuropathy.

It is estimated that up to 90 percent of people who undergo neuro-toxic chemotherapy will develop some level of peripheral neuropathy. So it is a serious side effect.[1] We have treated neuropathy in many cancer patients, and their results have been very good. To give you an idea of how each patient can be affected differently by peripheral neuropathy, I will relate the stories of two patients, Bob and Paula.

Bob was treated for cancer of the blood plasma cells (multiple myeloma) when he was 85-years-old, and he was in remission when he came to my office for a consultation. Initially, Bob was concerned because he had started to notice his feet were feeling extremely cold especially when he went to bed. That was his first sign of neuropathy, and he had no idea that this was the beginning of a disheartening complication. Bob initially thought he merely had cold feet, and he added an extra blanket to cover his feet at night. He had some improvement. His feet felt some warmer, but that was just for a short while, and then they felt cold again.

After several more days, Bob placed a little ceramic heater near his feet, covered his feet with the blanket and used that to keep them warm. The heater worked great for the first few days. After that, his feet were more than cold; they felt numb and as if they were frozen.

The intense cold sensation continued, and his feet became so painful and numb that Bob's walking and balance were very unsteady. Because Bob felt so unstable, he was anxious and afraid that he would fall, and his mobility was severely hampered. He was no longer able to do many jobs around his home, and he had to quit driving. He had always enjoyed taking his beloved dogs for rides on his scooter, but he had to stop. For Bob, that was a great loss.

Bob went to his oncologist about these new problems which started after his cancer treatments. His oncologist said, "There is nothing that can be done for you other than possibly trying one of the medications." The oncologist meant the group of drugs prescribed to try to treat the side effects of chemotherapy-induced peripheral neuropathy (CIPN). This would be drugs such as Lyrica, and Neurontin, or their generic versions. These drugs were originally FDA approved only for anti-seizure treatment but now, they are commonly prescribed for symptoms of neuropathy.

The drugs are of concern because there is great pressure from marketing to view the drugs as an alternative drug for pain syndromes. The oncologist also told Bob he could try Cymbalta, which is prescribed for anxiety and depression. However, each of the drugs noted can frequently have very serious side effects that include memory loss, euphoria, dizziness, addiction, and suicidal thoughts. Unfortunately, there are no long-term studies as to the effects of the drugs. Patients can experience withdrawal symptoms if they abruptly stop taking the drugs. Pregnant women should never take Lyrica, as it is the subject of lawsuits over congenital disabilities. Because of serious side effects, the manufacturers of these drugs are involved in significant lawsuits.

Bob tried all the recommended medical treatments including the medications prescribed and some physical therapy. He finally just gave up and was resigned to living his life with poor balance, pain, and numbness. That seemed better to him than what he had experienced as side effects from the medications.

Many doctors have not been trained in treatment other than allopathic (prescribing medications), and most are just not familiar with alternatives for treatment of peripheral neuropathy symptoms. However, there are treatment options for the symptoms of peripheral neuropathy besides potentially harmful drugs.

As you will read later, Bob had an amazing story, and it didn't come easy. You too don't have to live the rest of your life with pain and other debilitating symptoms. There is treatment available with the Busch Neuropathy Protocol™ - we don't only treat back and neck pain at the Busch Chiropractic Pain Center.

Another patient who suffered from neuropathy as a result of chemotherapy (CIPN) is Paula. Paula was 62 when we began treating her. Previously, she had been treated for colon cancer. Like Bob, Paula developed neuropathy after chemotherapy. So while chemotherapy drugs can save lives, they can also contribute to quality-of-life issues for some patients. As with many drugs there are trade-offs.

Paula's pain and discomfort were in her feet like Bob's symptoms, but her symptoms included a vice-like pressure in addition to the cold sensation as Bob had experienced. She also had painful feelings of 'pins and needles' in her hands and feet. Paula also talked with her oncologist about what she felt were significant problems. Her oncologist told her that she had neuropathy, and her chemotherapy medications caused it. This can be a "side effect of survival." The oncologist also told Paula that her symptoms were irreversible. Many doctors just don't know all the options for treating the symptoms of neuropathy following chemotherapy.

Very similar to Bob, Paula then experienced severe side effects from the medications prescribed to improve her neuropathy symptoms. She decided to stop taking them and look for alternative treatment options that didn't include more medication. She had tried anodyne therapy, an infrared treatment that has limitations and can burn patients.

Paula had no improvement. Because of this, she became very despondent thinking she would have to live the rest of her life limited and unable to do her normal activities while still suffering from loss of balance, constant discomfort and pain.

In addition to her neuropathy, Paula also suffered from severe low back pain and that restricted her from lifting or bending. Between her back, her feet and her hands, Paula was very limited in doing her regular work and daily activities like housekeeping, shopping, playing with her grandchildren or even watching her grandson play college baseball. She had serious balance problems that made it hard for her to get around. In short, her life was miserable.

After I did a comprehensive examination and a review of Paula's MRI, she was diagnosed with degenerative disc disease and spinal stenosis. She also had peripheral neuropathy in her feet and hands.

After beginning treatment with the DRS Protocol™ for her low back condition and combining her treatment with the Busch Neuropathy Protocol™ for the peripheral neuropathy in her hands and feet, Paula soon regained her normal mobility and balance. And she no longer suffered from the burning, tingling, and pain in her hands and feet.

Only occasionally did she have twinges in her feet and was able to get right back into her normal life's activities and work with little or no low back pain.

After treating, Paula could play with her grandchildren, and she frequently traveled to watch her grandson play baseball for a Division 1 college. As Paula improved, she saw her oncologist, and her oncologist was very happy and completely surprised with her recovery. He mentioned that her recovery was the only time he had ever seen a patient with CIPN symptoms improve.

These two patient histories, Bob and Paula, show differences between patients even when their neuropathy stems from essentially the same cause - chemotherapy. Each patient had individual situations, even though the cause was under one classification.   Therefore, it is common at my office, that neuropathy patients may be treated with combined treatment protocols, multiple therapies, and specific nutritional supplementation. To have successful outcomes, our bodies can only perform with what they are given, so we must treat the whole patient and not just the symptoms.

Infections can also cause peripheral neuropathy. Viruses and bacteria can attack nerve tissue, and these infections include shingles, Epstein-Barr virus, West Nile virus as well as herpes simplex viruses.

Some bacterial diseases that can affect the nerves include Lyme disease, diphtheria, and leprosy. While the last two are relatively rare in this country, Lyme disease is becoming increasingly common. Both Lyme disease and West Nile are spread by insects (ticks and mosquitoes respectively), and many people who are otherwise healthy can suddenly be riddled with nerve pain.

One other note about a virus most of us have never experienced, and that is polio. Polio has been eradicated in this country for decades, since the late seventies. What many forget is that millions of children in the 1950s survived the disease. Now those patients are older and are experiencing what has come to be known as post-polio syndrome. This syndrome, which only affects those who have previously had polio, includes loss of feeling and sensation in the legs and causes mobility problems and painful neuropathy.

HIV is a virus that causes AIDS and is associated with various forms of peripheral neuropathy. Thirty percent of those that have the disease will also experience peripheral neuropathy on some level.

Toxins can produce painful neuropathies, and there are several main categories. Of course, we've already mentioned chemotherapy, and yes it is a toxin. It has to be to kill cancer cells, so there are inevitable side effects. The same is true with any prescription or over-the-counter medicine like acetaminophen. All of which can be toxic in the right amounts.

Some anticonvulsant medications, as well as some heart and blood pressure medications, frequently can cause peripheral neuropathy. Common drugs prescribed for symptoms of neuropathy are actually anticonvulsants such as Lyrica, the generic name is pregabalin, and Neurontin, the generic name is gabapentin. Among their many side effects, they can cause numbness and tingling.

The Food and Drug Administration (FDA) recently announced a warning about very common antibiotics in the drug class of fluoroquinolones that can cause permanent peripheral neuropathy. This severe side effect has caused many of the antibiotics to be taken off the market. However, there are six FDA-approved drugs still being used at this time: ciprofloxacin, norfloxacin, ofloxacin, gemifloxacin, levofloxacin, and moxifloxacin .

The FDA now requires black box – most severe – warnings about peripheral neuropathy as a highly possible side effect to be listed in the inserts of each drug. Other possible side effects are ruptured tendons, retinal detachment, kidney failure and memory loss among others. The FDA is recommending against prescribing these drugs. If these medications must be taken, then it becomes a balancing act between prescribing the correct amount to achieve the desired outcome, and are the benefits worth the risk?

Toxins would also include agricultural and industrial chemicals, as well as home use, and household products such as pesticides and cleaners. We can also include medications, beauty products, artificial colorings and flavorings, and this is just a small part of the list. We are exposed to these items daily in this country, and it isn't hard for these chemicals to reach toxic levels; many toxins accumulate in the body. Again each person is different, and some people are extremely sensitive to toxins in the environment.

Certain occupations suffer much higher exposure to chemicals: painters, those who work in PVC/plastic manufacturing and in the rubber industry, chemical lab workers, farmers and those who work in printing among many other occupations

We can't leave out heavy metals that exist in our environment such as lead, mercury, and arsenic. People who work in factories are more highly exposed to industrial metals and chemicals. All of these can damage nerves depending on the degree of exposure, and there is no such thing as eliminating everything toxic from your environment or your life.

Often, patients who describe neuropathy symptoms will hear their doctors use the term 'idiopathic' neuropathy. That means 'no known cause.' They know a patient has pain and other problems, but it isn't known why, and there are times when an exact cause, or a combination of causes, will never be known. But that doesn't mean someone with idiopathic neuropathy can't find help.

Because neuropathy can be brought on by a number of factors, it can take some investigation and analysis to determine the cause, as each patient describes symptoms and conditions in different ways. Many patients come to me frustrated because other doctors they have seen including rheumatologists, neurologists, endocrinologists, dermatologists, podiatrist, infectious disease specialists, allergists, and immunologists may have concluded a diagnosis just on patients describing their symptoms. Therefore, many times neuropathy was misdiagnosed or not diagnosed at all.

Some doctors may even attribute symptoms to the patient just getting older, and they even go as far as to say the patient needs to "Learn to live with it," or "Nothing else can be done," or "Try this medication." This is when patients need to have patience and persistence.

Many patients expect to get a prescription for pain and discomfort when they see their medical doctor, and this is the most normal treatment path for a medical doctor to take. Conventional medical treatment options for the symptoms of peripheral neuropathy are largely centered on drug therapies such as antidepressants, anticonvulsants, steroids injections, lidocaine patches and pain pills. Many patients don't find the prescriptions help much, if at all, and they often develop additional symptoms and complaints.

Many of the drugs prescribed for neuropathy symptoms have warnings about side effects such as numbness, tingling, dizziness, and balance problems. These common side effects are some of the exact symptoms of neuropathy. Since falling is a leading cause of death for people over the age of seventy, taking a drug with major side effects of dizziness and balance problems is a potentially dangerous prescription.

However, some patients may request, or even demand, a specific drug without ever considering its side effects. The requests can be attributed to direct-to-consumer pharmaceutical advertising as seen on television; even though the medication's risks to its benefits are not made very clear.

Pharmaceutical advertising has created an expectation of some patients that the only answer to a health problem is a pill. Doctors prescribe, many times, as they feel pressured and concerned about not fulfilling patients' demands. If they do not, that can lead to unrealistic patients' dissatisfaction and poor practice reviews. While many people greatly benefit and even survive because of medications, government statistics show that over 70 percent of Americans are taking at least one prescription, 50 percent are taking two, and 15 percent are taking five or more. Older adults and a higher percentage of women are taking the most prescriptions.

However, most medical experts agree that 95 percent of the medications prescribed are not intended to treat underlying conditions that are the cause of patients' symptoms and that most drugs are for treating symptoms only and not the actual disease. In the case of treating peripheral neuropathy, the outcomes from drug therapy for symptoms are not very good.

As a doctor who treats symptoms of neuropathy, I understand the difficulties involved with diagnosing and treating. It requires a comprehensive examination and delving to get to the origin of the problem; as no two patients are the same. It is important to understand that symptoms caused by neuropathy can also have different patterns which can make a diagnosis even harder to pin down. For some patients, it starts suddenly, is intense for weeks or months and then gradually diminishes as the nerves become less symptomatic. For others, it is a slow progression from mild symptoms to gradually stronger symptoms over time. Changes could happen over a few years or even a couple of decades; it depends on the person.

Why Symptoms Vary So Much

Considering the complexity of our bodies, we still only understand a fraction of how the body works. This is particularly true in the case of nerve damage and pain treatment. Although science has achieved significant accomplishments and advances, there are still great gaps in knowledge and understanding, and much to learn.

The type of pain, organ dysfunction or decrease in mobility is directly related to the kind of nerve damage each patient experiences. To understand the various types of neuropathy, we first need to understand the types of nerves that are commonly affected. While there are many types of nerves, most can be grouped into three main categories: sensory, autonomic and motor.

Motor nerves control muscle movements which are necessary for walking, talking, writing or picking up objects. Damage to these nerves causes overall muscle weakness, painful cramps or twitching. Impaired nerves can also cause muscle atrophy and decreased reflexes, and loss of coordination between muscle groups. Patients with motor nerve damage may shuffle their feet or have their feet slapping on the floor because of foot drop. They may trip easily, drop coffee cups, or be too weak to do simple household chores.

Autonomic nerves are in charge of bodily functions that we don't consciously control such as digestion, breathing, and gland and heart function. The function of these nerves is incredibly complex, and symptoms often seem like normal age-related complaints such as constipation or diarrhea, urinary incontinence, and the inability to sweat or increased sweating. Patients may even have problems breathing or swallowing.

Sensory nerves control what sensations we feel and how we experience our world. This includes the ability to sense light touch and vibration, as well as hot and cold. Some patients say they feel as if they were wearing gloves or stockings all the time, and this is because the sensory nerves in their extremities have lost the ability to transmit fine senses.

When you consider these three areas of possible nerve damage and realize that patients rarely have damage to just one nerve group, it is easy to understand why there is such as a wide varying of symptoms from patient to patient. The damage among nerve groups can lead to tremendous frustration on the part of the patient, as treatment has to be the correct combination of therapies.

Frequently, a medical doctor's reflex response for treatment is to use the mainstream medical practices, and that is to generally default to medicate or operate. Alternative treatment is usually dismissed by mainstream medicine because they don't receive training in alternative or integrative treatments. So they are not familiar with alternative care and therefore really can't discuss alternative treatment options with their patients.

If a patient's symptoms are not severe, the doctor probably will look to immediately treating symptoms and may not delve too far into a cause. Patients rely on the doctor to fix their immediate problems – the symptoms. So, doctors treat by prescribing medications. Regrettably, the drugs are not always designed to treat the underlying condition causing the problem. Unfortunately, many patients are kept on multiple prescriptions for years, or even life-long dependency, without any hope of a cure or of resolving their underlying condition.

For medical billing and records, doctors must match a diagnostic code with a disease, (this is why everything is labeled a disease), and for many disease codes there are recommended courses of drug treatment. Prescribing drugs such as Lyrica and Neurontin is the attempt to treat only neuropathy symptoms since neuropathy has long been thought to be incurable.

The problem is some of the common side effects of these drugs range from behavioral changes like anxiety, depression, to a feeling of agitation, hostility, and restlessness. Some patients have even reported having muscle pain, weakness, memory problems, thoughts of suicide and even the same symptoms as their neuropathy. It seems the attempt at treatment is often worse than the original condition!

When we take any medication, there may be a trade-off. We are trading for what we hope will be the positive effects of a drug to make us feel better. However, there are times when the side effects become so hard to deal with that medications must be halted. Bad side effects are what happened to my patient Bob.

He tried all of the medications recommended by his medical doctors that were supposed to help his neuropathy symptoms. He quickly realized that he did not feel any better. In fact, most of the medications affected his personality and made him feel exhausted. Not only did the quality of his life suffer because of his symptoms of neuropathy, but also because of the side effects of his medications.

Bob told his wife if he couldn't get help he didn't want to live. His wife promised him she would find help for him, somehow somewhere. After being pushed and prodded by his wife, Bob finally decided to make an appointment with our office.

Once we confirmed Bob's diagnosis and thoroughly discussed the treatment recommendation of the Busch Neuropathy Protocol™, he began care immediately. After his first treatment, Bob finally slept straight through the night, and that hadn't happened in two years! After two weeks of treatment, he was able to walk, and his balance was back to normal. Bob was able to ride his scooter again and get outside with his dogs. This was what he really loved.

Bob came into the office after he began feeling better and joked that the reason he originally came for treatment was because his wife just plain pestered him into it. Now that he had experienced so much improvement, Bob looked forward to sticking around so his wife could pester him about other things for another couple of years. Bob had a great sense of humor and was a great guy who just wanted back the simple pleasures of his life – and he got them.

At my office, we do a comprehensive patient evaluation; it includes background questions, and sometimes these pose additional questions. One example of this is George. George was a type 2 diabetic. When I was asking questions about his background and job, George revealed that he delivered hazardous chemicals like acetylene and oxygen, and he had developed neuropathy about five years earlier. Of course, I immediately had to consider two possible causes for his neuropathy: diabetes, hazardous chemicals, or both. George made his appointment to be evaluated because there were times when he couldn't feel his feet. He had trouble feeling the truck pedals, which created a dangerous situation. Not only because he was driving a big truck, but because he was delivering toxic/explosive materials!

During George's initial examination, he discussed his previous efforts to get help. He had tried other treatments and had taken medications that affected his state of awareness. The drugs made him not only extremely tired but also he felt physically less stable. George stopped the prescriptions because he was concerned it might be dangerous for him to drive. Plus the drugs didn't help his neuropathy symptoms. He knew it was imperative to be alert and capable while driving a truck loaded with dangerous chemicals.

George treated with the Busch Neuropathy Protocol™, and one of the greatest outcomes for him was when he went on vacation and he drove comfortably to Florida. The feeling in his feet had returned, and when he walked on the beach, he could feel the sand between his toes for the first time in five years.

Another goal of George's was to walk on his treadmill and work out again. He had been afraid he would fall down and really hurt himself because he couldn't feel his feet and that was affecting his balance. So he had to stop walking and working out. After completing treatment with the Busch Neuropathy Protocol™, George was safely walking on his treadmill and working out. He had regained his balance and feeling, and he was very confident in his driving ability.

We treated George for many years, and he had no problems or exacerbations with his previous symptoms. It did not appear that his possible exposure to the dangerous chemicals played a role in the symptoms of neuropathy he developed, but that certainly could not have been completely ruled out. It is very satisfying for me to work with patients and see their long-lasting and positive outcomes. We aren't just treating pain, we are striving to restore our patients' quality of life.

Thirty Million People Suffer

The Foundation of Peripheral Neuropathy Association estimates that approximately thirty million people, in the U.S. suffer from peripheral neuropathy (PN): Causes are diabetes-60%, idiopathic, or unknown-23%, chemo-induced-10%, HIV/AIDS-2%, other-2%.[2] Yet many people have never heard of peripheral neuropathy. While not all symptoms may be eliminated, most peripheral neuropathy symptoms can be effectively managed to improve the quality of life for patients.

We have treated patients with the successful DRS Protocol™ for back and neck problems since 1996. While treating, we have seen many patients that are suffering from peripheral neuropathy and have tried everything including medications, painful testing, and other treatments: all without good outcomes. Without experiencing positive changes, this left the patients struggling and wandering down a road of endless disappointment.

Now we are able to address the pain and symptoms associated with peripheral neuropathy with the Busch Neuropathy Protocol™, a successful, noninvasive and drug-free approach. It has been exciting to see the changes patients experience. Many of our patients' primary care doctors and specialists have been pleased and surprised by the major improvements in their patients' condition after treating with the Busch Neuropathy Protocol™.

It is very common for family doctors, oncologists, and neurologist to refer patients to my clinic for evaluation, as there is no conflict in treatments and no worry about the interaction of drugs. It is a successful relationship, and now patients no longer need to suffer from the pain and symptoms that have restricted their lives.

A vital point I would encourage anyone reading this to know is that the sooner symptoms are treated, the better the outcome. Not only can symptoms of peripheral neuropathies be treated, patients often regain their normal and active lives.

Dr. Richard Busch III

Seeing that my patients experience such positive changes in their lives and watching them gain in their relationships with their family and friends is extremely rewarding for my patients and me, as their doctor.

Treatment with the Busch Neuropathy Protocol™ can give patients a new lease on life, and many times reduces or eliminates the need for prescription pain medications and other drugs. A good goal for patients is to be able to get off of medications that can affect them both physically and mentally. The Busch Neuropathy Protocol™ is noninvasive and drug-free; there is absolutely no concern about drug interactions. The protocol is safe, and it works.

Dr. Richard Busch III

CHAPTER 7
Diabetic Neuropathy

CHAPTER 7
Diabetic Neuropathy

I feel it is important to separate diabetic neuropathy from other types of peripheral neuropathy, as people with diabetes are the largest group (60%) of patients affected by neuropathy. Over 30 million people have diabetes in the US, and in the U.S., another individual is newly diagnosed with diabetes every 21 seconds (4,110 people today)! [1]

Having type I diabetes means that your body does not produce insulin at all. Causes of type 1 diabetes are not altogether understood. It is known that a genetic component can be part of the cause, along with the body becoming autoimmune - the immune system attacks and destroys insulin-producing cells in the pancreas.

Some studies suggest a virus may trigger the body to target its pancreas. Type 2 diabetes happens when the pancreas does not produce enough insulin, or the body is insulin resistant which means the cells do not accept or respond to the normal effect of insulin.

Type I diabetes was named juvenile diabetes, as the onset was usually in childhood. With type 1 diabetes, the patients are one hundred percent insulin dependent their entire lives. Type 2 is the most prevalent type of diabetes and previously was referred to as 'late onset' diabetes, as it was diagnosed much later in life – often when a person reached 40 or 50 years old. However, today even teens and individuals in their twenties are being diagnosed with type 2 diabetes. Lifestyle factors such as diet and weight and genetics are strong contributing factors to type 2 diabetes. Now almost 40% percent of Americans, including young people and adults, are obese.[2] They are obese for many reasons like diet, food additives, bad fats, hormones and antibiotics given to animals we eat, genetics and lack of exercise. With all these factors, diabetes seems to show itself much earlier.

Current estimates are that 30.3 million people have diabetes (9.4% of the US population) and 84.1 million adults (33.9% of the adult US population), 18 years and older, are borderline diabetics or have the condition known as prediabetes and 15-30 percent of those who are prediabetic will develop diabetes within five years.[3] This information is extremely relevant because a high number of peripheral neuropathy cases are the result of uncontrolled, or poorly managed, diabetes.

High blood sugar is considered an extreme metabolic disorder and absolutely must be controlled effectively. Many people may think of excessive blood sugar as relatively harmless, yet it can cause catastrophic problems if left untreated. Elevated blood sugar leads to diabetic nerve damage or peripheral neuropathy which causes numbness, loss of sensation and sometimes chronic pain in the extremities.

Many people with diabetes lose feeling in their hands and feet to the point they can no longer feel injuries or wounds. Infections and complications can cause open wounds leading to extended hospital stays and even amputation. Peripheral neuropathy is one of the most common complications of diabetes and can also cause problems with internal organs. The heart, digestive tract and sexual organs can be affected. This can lead to indigestion, diarrhea/constipation, dizziness, and impotence. It is easy to see why peripheral neuropathy can also lead to depression.

It is estimated that close to 60-70 percent of diabetics will be plagued with peripheral neuropathy.[4] This is an extremely high number, and given the total number of people in the US with diabetes, it is understandable why they make up the majority of our peripheral neuropathy patients. Just as other patients, everyone experiences different symptoms with diabetic neuropathy. Some initially have no symptoms at all, some experience pain or tingling, while others go completely numb. Some experience sharp stabbing pain, while others feel pinching or vibrating. Others will have dizziness, faintness, and loss of balance. Because diabetes is a long-term illness, many patients don't notice their symptoms gradually getting worse.

A patient of mine named Susan was a 65-year-old type I diabetic, and she really loved to travel in her RV and camp. Susan enjoyed almost any outdoor activity. Her problem was the severe pain that she had developed in her feet from neuropathy. She could not go camping or hiking, and she could not garden and do yard work because she could not tolerate her severe foot pain long enough to do the smallest job. She couldn't handle the pain for even a few minutes. Susan also had trouble with her gait and balance, and she was afraid of falling and seriously getting hurt. She had come close to falling many times.

After a thorough evaluation in our office, it was determined that Susan did have peripheral neuropathy in her feet, and that was the cause of her foot pain. This limited her ability to stand and walk. She also had problems with sensations like hot and cold, as well as a burning pain in her feet. Susan had trouble sensing light touch and an overall muscle weakness. Her neuropathy had progressed much further than many of our other patients. She was quite debilitated, and the pain made it very hard for her to sleep.

Within her first week of treatment, Susan's foot pain had majorly improved. She was already walking much better, and of great importance, she was able to sleep through the night. Shortly thereafter, she was camping again and started traveling. Susan continued to travel, camp, and do all the things that she wanted to do with little to no numbness or pain in her feet. She had recovered her balance and made a remarkable recovery.

As with other types of peripheral neuropathy, the symptoms of diabetic neuropathy are often worse at night, and because diabetes can affect many nerves, patients will often have many multifaceted symptoms. They can experience a heightened sensitivity to touch when something as light as a bed sheet can cause excruciating pain. They may have difficulty moving or coordinating muscle groups, which cause them to be unable to get up from a chair, grasp a cup or fork, or even write their name. As the body tries to adapt to the increasing nerve damage, the patient may feel progressively unable to balance, stand still or walk unaided.

Because type 2 diabetics often have multiple health issues, it is not uncommon for peripheral neuropathy to go undiagnosed. Or, even if neuropathy is diagnosed, it may be treated as a low priority until it is well advanced. While damage may be gradual in diabetic patients, it is cumulative. The quicker neuropathy is diagnosed and treated the better the long-term outcome will be.

Another patient, Greg, was a 72-year-old man who developed peripheral neuropathy as a result of either his type 2 diabetes or from his statin drug prescription that his medical doctor had prescribed for his elevated cholesterol or both. Greg had been complaining about neuropathy symptoms for about nine months before visiting my office. However, there is no telling exactly how long his neuropathy had been developing. His symptoms became severe enough for him to look for help. This is not unusual for diabetic neuropathy patients because neuropathy is just one of many of their health problems.

Greg really enjoyed riding and maintaining his motorcycle. He also was very good at carpentry and woodworking, and he spent long hours in his shop working on different projects. Because neuropathy developed in both Greg's hands and his feet, he had a lot of trouble with woodworking and working on his motorcycle. In fact, he had to completely stop woodworking because he almost cut off his thumb and had to have surgery. He said he didn't feel anything when the saw blade sliced his thumb. He had lost that much feeling in his hands.

Like Susan, Greg had trouble going to sleep and staying asleep due to the numbness, tingling and burning sensations that developed. Neuropathy can, in many cases, be so uncomfortable that the patient cannot get comfortable enough to fall asleep. The anxiety that comes from insomnia and the brain fog that develops in some of these patients with sleep deprivation can be very debilitating and can make the patient dread bedtime and night-time.

Greg improved quickly from treatment with the Busch Neuropathy Protocol™ and began sleeping well. He regained almost total sensation in his feet and his hands. He was able to safely use his saws and other woodworking equipment. He bought a trike assembly for his motorcycle, and he did the installation on his own. Because he had regained the feeling in his hands and feet, Greg was able to resume enjoying his life of woodworking as well as riding and working on his motorcycle.

For anyone who is diabetic, even those who don't feel they have symptoms of diabetic neuropathy yet, it pays to be vigilant. Of course, the best thing you can do is keep your blood sugar levels under control all the time – not just sometimes. I'm always amazed at the number of people with diabetes who don't seem to realize how much control they have over avoiding future complications of diabetes simply by keeping their blood sugar well monitored and following an appropriate diet.

Don't Wait to See a Doctor

If you are noticing basic symptoms of neuropathy such as burning, tingling, pain, and weakness in your hands or feet, or balance problems, or dizziness don't wait to see your doctor. Even a small cut or sore on your foot can be dangerous and can easily become infected and turn into an ulcer. If left untreated infected sores can turn into gangrene; a condition that will require surgery and even amputation. Don't wait, the earlier you are diagnosed and treated the better the prospects are for controlling your symptoms and avoiding more severe problems.

Another of my patients we helped was Barbara. At the time, Barbara was a 66-year-old type 2 diabetic. She had been diabetic for about 15 years, but unfortunately, she had not done the best job of following recommendations for diet or exercise. She felt she had been pretty active on her farm and that was enough. However, when she finally came to my office, Barbara was taking Metformin for blood sugar and gabapentin for her neuropathy symptoms of numbness, tingling, and sharp shooting pain in both her hands and feet.

The neuropathy had tremendously slowed her down. Soon after she began treatment with the Busch Neuropathy Protocol™, she began to talk about going for nice long walks and traveling to Chicago to walk and shop on Michigan Avenue. She was very excited about getting back to her work on the farm and being able to catch up on her chores.

Obviously, Barbara's neuropathy had been affecting her ability to perform the activities that she needed to do and really enjoyed. As a result, she had gotten behind with her farm work and had stopped traveling completely. Her peripheral neuropathy, which was caused by her diabetes, had dramatically affected her quality of life.

By treating with the Busch Neuropathy Protocol™ she saw wonderful changes, and Barbara completely regained her ability to keep up with her normal activities. However, she knew she had to make some manageable lifestyle modifications like changing her diet and monitoring blood sugar levels carefully.

Barbara was not only very interested in losing weight, but she really wanted to get off of her medications. As a result of putting Barbara on a diet and the proper supplementation, she lost 60 pounds. The weight loss enabled her to get off of her diabetes and neuropathy medications with her doctor's approval, and she regained her normal lifestyle. It was amazing to see the results and the differences that she had made for her own life.

There are many preventative actions a diabetic can take to take care of themselves. I urge my patients to carefully watch their diets, and I encourage exercise. I also recommend that everyone with diabetes inspect their feet daily. If that is too difficult, have someone help you, or you can use a mirror. Always wear comfortable shoes. Tight shoes can cause sores. Wash and dry your feet completely and then use lotions, but not between the toes, to avoid cracking. See a podiatrist to cut your toenails - do not go to a salon.

It is important to have your doctor do a foot exam, as well. If you detect a scrape or sore, do not try to treat it yourself. Contact your medical doctor right away and get treatment. The goal is to stop a small problem from becoming severe.

Inspecting your feet daily may seem like a lot of checking, however, if your feet are numb, or beginning to have numbness, you may not realize you are developing a sore or skin ulcer. Pain gets our attention and is an indicator that something is wrong, but not feeling pain is also an indicator and patients should be on high alert.

Another neuropathy patient we treated was John. When I first met John, he was a terrified 80-year-old gentleman with type 2 diabetes. His legs and feet were very swollen, and he had suffered for six months with an open wound on the bottom of his foot.

For those who have diabetes, little scrapes and cuts can quickly become ulcers. Wounds and ulcers can be very slow to heal, if at all. Ulcers are prevalent in patients that have developed peripheral arterial disease (PAD), and many diabetics develop PAD. PAD is a disease where plaque builds up and narrows the arteries which in turn limits blood flow and oxygenation to the legs, feet and other areas of the body. PAD may cause pain, numbness and tingling in the legs and feet.

Because of the diminished blood flow there can be pooling of fluids, and this can cause the breakdown of soft tissue and skin. This pooling can produce ulcers. Even poor-fitting shoes can cause skin ulcers. Patients that have diabetes often get nerve damage or peripheral neuropathy due to high blood sugar that has damaged their peripheral nerves. This damage can stop the feeling in the feet and hands. Therefore, patients' often don't realize when they are injured from burns, cuts, bruises, and abrasions. A small injury can turn out to be a disaster.

The problem with ulcers and injuries is slow and poor quality healing. This can lead to the breakdown of the skin and over time, too much damage takes place. All this invites the risk of bacterial infection. There can be a point when the body cannot recover, and the only option then becomes amputation.

Some other complicating factors of diabetic wounds can include gangrene, which is caused by loss of adequate blood supply, and it does progress quickly if it is not correctly treated. In dealing with these wounds, the order of treatment goes from keeping the wound clean and dressed with antibiotics for stopping the spread of infection to debridement, which means removing wounded and dead tissue.

Many times when a patient has wounds and or ulcers, they are referred to wound care specialists and finally amputation. The wound and infection get to the point that they can no longer be healed with conventional care.

This is what almost happened to our patient John. The traditional care he had been receiving was not helping, and there was the recommendation of amputation. The wound on the bottom of John's foot was the size of a silver dollar, raw, oozing and very dangerous. John had treated for a long time at a wound center, but the wound would not heal. His medical doctor had said the next step was amputation. John met with a surgeon, and the surgeon agreed that amputation was the only way to control John's wound problem.

John told me the reason he was in my office was that he would do everything he could before having his foot cut off. He was concerned about even living through the surgery. If he did survive would he fully recover, and would he ever be able to get around? For John, it was not just the quantity of his life, but the quality of his life.

We began John's treatment with the Busch Neuropathy Protocol™, and within a month his foot wound was almost completely healed. He continued to improve until his wound had fully healed. When John saw his medical doctor for a regular appointment, his doctor was completely shocked to see John's major improvements and that his wound had actually healed. John got back to sleeping great, walking with much more motivation and confidence, and back to his normal life.

I have been treating patients since 1996, and many of them are very special and humorous. As was Dorothy, a wonderful lady, who was 104 at the time. Once I asked her what she thought had caused her discomfort. She quickly looked at me and said; "Honey, I'm 104-years old. Just getting out of my bed in the morning causes me great discomfort!"

Each patient is at a different stage in life, and what can be a normal activity for one patient may be a greater challenge for another. As people age, they experience different levels of independence and activity. Certainly John was no different. He regained much of the activity that he had lost due to his foot wound. He was able to return to his regular tasks like mowing his lawn and taking out the garbage. We saw John on a monthly basis, and he had sustained his improvement.

John had talked with me about how distressed he had been even thinking about having an amputation. He felt that at his age of 80 he could never imagine going through the pain and emotional trauma from having an amputation as well as the long-term rehabilitation that would be necessary.

John told me that he knew he was an older man, and he didn't want to spend any of his life going through the agony and recovery from an amputation. Needless to say, John was grateful that he had finally found the right care that healed his foot wound. John said he was elated that when it was his time he was "taking all of his parts" with him, although he didn't plan on that happening soon because he had too much to do.

Patients with diabetic neuropathy are, and will continue to be, a large part of our peripheral neuropathy practice. Peripheral neuropathy and its symptoms are not correctable by drugs or surgery. It is good news that now there is a successful treatment, the Busch Neuropathy Protocol™, to slow down or even reverse a patient's immobility, pain and other symptoms of neuropathy.

This specialized treatment protocol is drug-free and pain-free. It involves multiple treatment elements including laser therapy, vibration therapy, specific nutritional supplementation, and the state-of-the-art infrared light therapy. This therapy has long been well recognized internationally, and these recent advancements offer hope for many more to live more pain-free and enjoyable lives.

I have found the highest personal satisfaction and pride in my professional career by being able to develop and implement treatment protocols that are drug-free, noninvasive and successful.

I have seen that there is greater gain and healing when there is a strong patient-doctor relationship. By implementing our patient-centered healthcare approach, we are able to address numerous issues, encourage our patients to assume healthier behaviors, and at the same time bring relief and healing to hurting patients.

Don't wait to find help if you have symptoms of peripheral neuropathy, because you can be helped. Obviously, the best treatment is prevention, but if you have been diagnosed with neuropathy or have symptoms you are at risk, and you should seek help from a qualified doctor.

Dr. Richard Busch III

CHAPTER 8
Nutrition and Fitness

CHAPTER 8
Nutrition and Fitness

When dealing with patients experiencing chronic pain, there are many questions that need to be asked, and some of those involve a topic that many people try to avoid: diet. A little-known fact for patients who experience pain is that there are some things they can do nutritionally to help decrease inflammation and, as a result, experience less pain.

There are many schools of thought regarding nutrition—far too many to cover here. I am primarily focusing on some standard ideas, and I will leave the debate about the perfect diet to another book. After all, this is not about the perfect diet; this is about improvement.

When a new patient is evaluated, a history of medications, supplements, over-the-counter pain relievers, and other remedies is compiled. Information is gathered about overall nutritional habits. In certain cases, when a patient has had a severe long-term problem, the assessment must go deeper. I need to look into the regular dietary habits to determine how much protein, fat, and carbohydrates are consumed. Many doctors do not relate a disc condition to the subject of nutrition and digestion, but there is a compelling reason for this line of inquiry. Many back and neck problems, along with headaches, can be related to systemic inflammation caused by diet, a lifestyle of alcohol and tobacco use, and the inability to absorb or digest nutrients.

Patients who have continuing problems of indigestion, constipation, or diarrhea rarely think of these as serious. However, these are symptoms of underlying problems. Usually, these problems do not send people to the doctor before serious complications begin, and they commonly use over-the-counter (OTC) products to deal with them.

Using these products, in addition to pain relievers, becomes a means of continuing to self-medicate. Some offer relief, but they cannot correct conditions that have been disguised for years. A good example of an OTC remedy is an antacid, which may interact with medications. Many medications warn against the use of antacids. Additionally, some antacids will contain aluminum or a large amount of sodium, and they may create a laxative effect or cause constipation.

Cause and Effect

Some foods will directly contribute to inflammation as well as the pain from inflammation. This not only slows the patient's response to care but can also serve to discourage the patient. The food we eat—or do not eat—affects how our bodies function. We need a variety of foods to be able to heal properly and quickly. Some patients who have greater difficulty with healing are those with dietary restrictions or poor diets in general.

While you may think that this does not apply to you, prepackaged food, especially junk food, has been through extensive processing that destroys its nutritional value. Highly refined products such as white flour, white sugar, and white rice are stripped of most nutritional content. Processing will remove much of the flavor and change the appearance of food. This problem is fixed by adding artificial flavors and colors. Some flavorings are actually chemicals and are used because they are cheaper than real flavors. Because food needs to be shipped long distances and have a long shelf life, preservatives are added. Hormones and antibiotics are added to beef, chicken, and milk sold to the public, and the effects of these on the human body have hardly been considered. Preservatives and pesticides can have cumulative and detrimental effects on our bodies, and processed foods lose most of their vitamins, minerals, enzymes during the preservation process.

Stay Close to Nature

Whole foods that are closest to their natural form are best for our bodies. They are not overly processed or adulterated with an excess of salt, sugar, additives, and fat. Foods that supply most nutrients are whole grains, fish, fruit, and vegetables. In today's hurried world, people eat a diet of fast food, junk food, and prepackaged food, without realizing that they are inhibiting their body's ability to heal and increasing inflammation.

Most do not understand what nutrients the body needs. Popular diets may convince them that certain elements of foods are "bad," leading them to avoid those items. Many different foods are necessary for good health. I have listed a few of the more essential in this chapter.

While this is by no means a complete list, it will give you an idea of how a lack of these items affects your body and why it is important to be educated about proper nutrition.

A Tale of Two Carbs

Research is increasingly turning attention to the consequences of poor and inadequate digestion as the source of chronic degenerative problems such as myofibrosis and arthritis.

As with all foods, there are desirable elements and less desirable elements. Contrary to popular belief, all carbohydrates are not an enemy. There are good carbohydrates and bad carbohydrates. Carbohydrates are a main source of energy for our bodies. There are three kinds of carbohydrates: fiber, sugars, and starches. The body will use some carbohydrates for immediate energy, while converting others to fat to use later.

Carbohydrates have gotten a bad rap in the news and in the minds of the general population because of the easy availability of simple carbohydrates. Simple carbohydrates are abundant in fast food, junk food, and a whole variety of "foods", all which are low in fiber, that have nothing in common with the food humans consumed prior to the last 50-plus-years. These include chips, sodas, lattes, and pretty much anything found in the "snack" aisle of the grocery store.

Many diet programs urge the reduction or even elimination of carbohydrates from the diet. However, carbohydrates are used by the body exclusively for energy. A diet that excludes carbohydrates can produce side effects such as weakness, brain fog, constipation, and stiffness in the joints. Complex carbohydrates are actually a necessary part of a balanced diet. They are very important in the production of energy, and they are found in the following foods:

• wheat germ
• bran
• barley
• maize
• buckwheat
• cornmeal
• oatmeal
• brown rice
• pasta
• whole grain breads
• muesli
• root vegetables, such as potatoes and yams
• squash
• peas
• lentils
• corn

These foods are good sources of complex carbohydrates. When consumed in as close to a natural state as possible; they are wonderful sources of energy for the body. This is not a complete list of complex carbohydrates, just a good starting point. Eating foods in their simplest, organic form will provide the most benefits.

When treating disc-related conditions, a main objective is to reduce inflammation, so the nerves and tissue can recover.

Simple carbohydrates interfere with that process. Simple carbohydrates not only contribute to weight gain and are empty calories, some can contribute to the inflammatory process of the body, and that can slow healing which makes the patient less responsive to care.

Protein

Protein from animal sources has been shunned by those who espouse a vegetarian philosophy. Normal sources of protein in a regular diet include red meat, poultry, fish, and eggs. Protein is also found in plant products, dairy, legumes, nuts, and seeds. These foods should be part of a well-rounded diet. Skin, bones, muscles, and organs contain protein.

Protein is in the blood, hormones, and enzymes. The body needs a little bit of everything to be healthy. A diet low in protein is also often deficient in iron, zinc, thiamin, and vitamin B6. Protein is a major building block in the amino acids of the body and plays a considerable role in cellular function. Glucose is also obtained from protein. It is absorbed more slowly into the bloodstream and does not cause a rapid increase in blood sugar.

Unlike glucose, the body does not store much protein, and if it becomes deficient in protein, this will cause the muscle to break down, much in the same manner as when people starve.

While vegetarians and vegans avoid meat, they still need protein for their bodies to function correctly. Protein is an essential building block that helps create cells and assists in the healing process. While almost all vegetarian and vegan diet programs stress the need to seek sources of protein other than animal sources, it can be challenging to consume enough protein.

Many patients I treat are vegetarians, and some of them tend to be protein-deficient. Many vegetarians eat soy-based products and soybeans. While these are high in protein, they also include phytoestrogens, which can have unintended effects—especially in post-menopausal women. Phytoestrogens have been shown to contribute to bone loss and increase the risk of vertebral fractures. In children, phytoestrogens can cause early menses and other developmental changes.

Even if you choose not to include soy products in your diet, there are other natural sources of protein, such as nuts and sweet potatoes. Below is a partial list (the amounts are for one-cup portions) and a comparison with the amounts of protein found in examples of meat sources:

Non-meat Sources

- lentils (18 grams of protein)
- black beans (15 grams)
- kidney beans (13 grams)
- chickpeas (12 grams)
- vegetarian baked beans (12 grams)
- pinto beans (12 grams)
- black-eyed peas (11 grams)
- peas (9 grams)
- spinach (5 grams)
- broccoli (4 grams)

Meat Sources

- 4 ounces chicken breast (35 grams of protein)
- 3 ounces beef (26 grams)
- 3 ounces turkey (25 grams)
- 3 ounces salmon (23 grams)

These are a few examples of protein sources. I would encourage anyone to research various sources of protein and to make certain to consume enough to support their body and maintain good health.

Fat

Fats are not automatically the enemy. They help the body absorb vitamins, maintain the structure and function of cells, and help maintain the immune system. Fats provide the energy and help create an energy reserve. Fats also help maintain consistent body temperature. They are also involved in the production and regulation of steroids within the body.

"Fat is bad," has become a popular mantra for the food industry over the past couple of decades. Food products now tout reduced fat, low fat, or no fat. In our quest to control weight and improve health, marketers have learned that by producing and promoting products with less fat, they increase sales. However, fat is an essential element in constructing and maintaining cell membrane, and fat aids the body in absorbing essential vitamins.

Without enough of the right kind of fat, cells cannot function as well, and this includes the cells of the nervous system, which includes the spinal cord. The right kind of fat is required for good health.

What is the right kind of fat? Good fats are the omega-3 fatty acids. Some easy to find sources of omega-3 fatty acids are walnuts, flaxseed, beans, fish, olive oil, squash, and cold-water fish. Omega-3 fats help limit inflammation by producing certain chemicals in the body that will aid in controlling inflammation. These chemicals will reduce (or, more correctly, inhibit) inflammation.

Fats to avoid include any hydrogenated fats, such as saturated and trans fats, and oils derived from corn or cottonseed. While eating products light in fat is not a bad course of action, especially if you trying to watch your weight, you have to be aware that some fat is required for health. Studies now show that even butter in moderate amounts is healthy, although using olive oil would be preferred.

One item of note when discussing fat is cholesterol. Cholesterol cannot dissolve in the blood. It has to be transported to and from the cells by carriers called lipoproteins. There are two types of cholesterol. Low-density lipoprotein, or LDL, is known as "bad" cholesterol. High-density lipoprotein, or HDL, is known as "good" cholesterol.

These two types of lipids, along with triglycerides and Lp(a) cholesterol, make up your total cholesterol count, which can be determined through a standard blood test.

When too much LDL cholesterol is in the blood, it can build up on the walls of the arteries and form plaque—a hard deposit that can narrow the arteries and make them less flexible—which is a condition known as atherosclerosis. If a clot forms and blocks a narrowed artery, a heart attack or stroke can result.

About one-fourth to one-third of blood cholesterol is carried by high-density lipoprotein (HDL). HDL cholesterol is known as "good" cholesterol because high levels seem to protect against heart attack, while low levels increase the risk of heart disease.

Medical experts think that HDL carries cholesterol away from the arteries and back to the liver, where it is passed from the body. Some experts believe that HDL removes excess cholesterol from arterial plaque, slowing its buildup.

Triglyceride is a form of fat made in the body. The causes of elevated triglycerides can include obesity, physical inactivity, smoking, excess alcohol consumption, and a diet very high in carbohydrates (60% or more of total calories).

People with high triglycerides often have a high total cholesterol level, including a high LDL level and a low HDL level. Many people with heart disease or diabetes also have high triglyceride levels.

I am often asked about specific types of synthetic fats, such as margarine, which was promoted as heart-healthy for years. However, margarine contains large amounts of trans fats from hydrogenated oils.

My stance is that if it does not occur in nature or by pressing something natural, such as olives or coconut, then you should probably not eat it. Eat organically or as close to the natural source as possible.

Anti-Inflammatory Foods

Many good food choices will help decrease pain from inflammation:

Vegetables
- bok choy
- broccoli
- brussels sprouts
- cabbage
- cauliflower
- chard
- collards
- garlic
- green beans
- green onions/spring onions
- kale
- leeks
- olives
- spinach
- sweet potatoes

Fruits

- apples
- avocados
- black currants
- blueberries
- kiwi fruit
- lemons
- limes
- oranges
- papaya
- pineapple (fresh)
- raspberries
- rhubarb
- strawberries
- cherries

Protein

- beef (lean organic)
- chicken breast (skinless, boneless, and organic)
- oysters
- rainbow trout
- salmon
- snapper
- striped bass
- whitefish

Oils

- avocado
- coconut
- olive

There is some indication that plants in the nightshade family can increase inflammation in the body. These plants include tomatoes, eggplant, peppers, and potatoes. These plants contain a substance called solanine, which may increase inflammation and pain in certain people. The best course of action is to eliminate this category from the diet for two weeks and then reintroduce it to see if pain and inflammation increases.

Hydration

Few people drink enough water. I do not mean liquid. Many people drink coffee, sodas, tea, or other drinks all day, but they do not drink enough water. The problem is compounded by the fact that many of these other drinks can have adverse effects on a person's health.

Our bodies are made up of 70% water, and water is necessary for the body to function. Humans can live without food for literally weeks. Without water, we would last a few days to a week at most. Dehydration compounds any health issue by preventing the cells from getting enough fluid to function properly and by reducing the body's ability to eliminate waste. When the body is dehydrated, cellular waste builds up in the tissue, rather than being carried out of the body via the kidneys.

Proper hydration is critical for recovery for any condition. Not only does it help clear away the results of cellular metabolism (i.e., waste), it is also very important for many other cellular reactions as well. Fluid is important for cellular function.

The majority of my patients I talk with believe they are drinking enough water, but this is rarely the case. A good rule is to drink 8-10, 8-ounce glasses a day, or more when exercising or in a hot environment. That adds up to 64-80 ounces a day. I recommend that a patient fill a pitcher with the amount of water they should drink each day and then drink that amount. They are surprised how much water it really is and quickly realize they are under-hydrating their bodies. The joints of the spine and the discs rely on the hydraulic properties of water and the hydration of the cartilage for proper function as well as the ability to heal.

Many elderly patients may limit their fluid intake because of their physical problems and limitations, such as arthritis, Alzheimer's, and stroke. The thirst sensation can diminish, and it may be difficult for them to drink enough water. The elderly, or anyone suffering from incontinence, may deliberately limit their fluid intake. All this plays a role in dehydration.

Health issues can be exacerbated by caffeine, which can cause restlessness, anxiety, irritability, tremors, sleeplessness, headaches, gastrointestinal symptoms, and abnormal heart rhythms. In some individuals, caffeine can increase blood pressure. Some people are extra-sensitive to even small amounts of caffeine and can have headaches as a result.

Low back pain can be exacerbated by caffeine. Many people cannot make it through their day without sodas and coffee. These can create inflammation, and they stress the kidneys.

Kidney stress/disease can cause low back pain that mimics other conditions. Caffeine, which is a mild diuretic, can interfere with mineral absorption and utilization. There are also serious side effects from the aspartame in diet drinks and sugar-free products. Aspartame should be avoided!

Vitamins, Minerals and Enzymes

As an important part of each treatment protocol, I provide specific professional-line supplementation to my patients. There are numerous vitamins and minerals that are essential in helping your body heal. Vitamin C is one of the most well-known. It is water-soluble and is not stored in the body. Vitamin C is essential in the formation of collagen. Therefore, it is an important part of the spinal disc. It is also an important component of blood vessels, tendons, ligaments, and bone. In addition to the spinal discs, the tissues that most require vitamin C are bone, scar tissue, and blood vessels. These tissues contain a large amount of collagen. Therefore, vitamin C is significant in the treatment of disc related conditions. Vitamin C deficiency can contribute to poor wound healing and weak and irregular scar tissue formation.

It is important to include B vitamins, especially B6 (pyridoxine), which is involved in more bodily functions than any other vitamin. B6 benefits both physical and mental health. It aids in breaking down protein and helps maintain healthy red blood cells, the nervous system, and the immune system. B6 is also a vital part of producing neurotransmitters, the chemicals that allow the brain and nerves to communicate. It also is beneficial for nerve compression conditions and arthritis. In many ways, B6 helps the nerves heal. B6 has been used for many years as an adjunct to the treatment of carpal tunnel syndrome. All B vitamins are water-soluble and are instrumental in supporting growth, development, and chemical reactions in the body. They are also an important part of turning food into energy. When a person is under stress, it is important to supplement with B vitamins.

A balanced diet that includes lean meats, grain products, vegetables, and fruits should be adequate to supply all the B vitamins needed. However, since most people do not eat a sufficient balanced diet, there is a definite need to supplement the B vitamins.

I often recommend calcium, the most abundant mineral found in the body, and magnesium, which works in tandem with calcium. Together they play a vital role in maintaining healthy bones and a healthy nervous system. People who eat large amounts of processed foods (with most, the magnesium is removed) are not getting enough magnesium in their diets.

Calcium makes up 99% of bones and teeth, and it plays a major part in maintaining the bones. Calcium and magnesium affect the nervous system and function as natural tranquilizers. They are both sleep aids, in addition to preventing muscle spasms. It is common for patients who live in pain from disc-related problems to have a heightened sense of pain associated with muscle spasms. Calcium and magnesium help reduce the pain and calm the spasms, which in turn will help patients sleep more comfortably and readily. Other supplementations are also important in the healing process of the disc and cartilage.

It is important to understand that the body uses vitamins and minerals with the help of enzymes. Enzymes in the body are catalysts, and most are a class of protein. The purpose of enzymes is to facilitate chemical reactions, such as the breaking down of protein. This function is dependent on a substance called protease, which is an enzyme that specifically aids in the breaking down of protein.

Enzymes should occur naturally in the food we eat and allow us to break down nutritional substances so they can be fully used by our bodies. Without these enzymes, the nutritional value is lost. The best source of enzymes is food in its natural form that has been grown in healthy conditions. In order to preserve foods by canning or other methods to allow for shipping and storage, enzymes are destroyed by food processing and manufacturing.

Therefore, the more food is processed, the less the body is able to derive proper nutrients. When patients are enzyme deficient, they frequently suffer from chronic digestive disorders.

Because the body has difficulty breaking down food, referred pain may be experienced. Remember, referred pain is pain that is felt in a different place in the body other than the source. For example, with the gallbladder or heart, pain manifests in another area, such as the left shoulder or arm for the heart, or the right elbow or shoulder for the gallbladder. There is a host of reflex patterns throughout the body. These are a result of muscle spasm and nerve irritation because there is stress on the body or organ system that corresponds to certain reflex points/patterns. Often, patients who experience chronic degenerative conditions and have these referral patterns will benefit from enzyme therapy.

Enzyme replacement therapy, the art and science of using nutrition to maintain homeostasis and health in the body, was pioneered by a colleague of mine, Dr. Howard Loomis. He is the founder and president of Enzyme Formulations, Inc. Dr. Loomis trains and certifies doctors to evaluate patients through a physical examination process, blood tests, and a 24-hour urinalysis. A patient that I would test is one who is slow to respond to care or has reached a plateau in progress, or a patient with a very chronic condition and other chronic complaints such as fatigue, headache, and digestive disturbances. These patients may have problems breaking down protein or may be protein-deficient. This type of patient can easily be tested for an underlying nutritional or digestive problem. This problem can be addressed with enzyme replacements, which in many cases easily stabilizes the patient's condition.

I often see patients with chronic lumbar disc conditions, a situation in which their spine or pelvis will never completely stabilize. This type of patient describes the problem as if something in the back or pelvis "just goes out." These patients will benefit from an enzyme, TRCTN. The purpose of TRCTN is to provide a source of vitamins and minerals from protein nutritive herbs combined with enzymes.

I have found that this product helps the patient's pelvis stabilize, and I like to call it the "pelvic stabilizer." If the patient's problem is related to spinal nerve damage or irritation and the spine does not stabilize, then the patient should benefit from CMPRS. The purpose of CMPRS is to provide a source of vitamins and minerals from alternative, lymphatic, and diuretic herbs. I refer to this as the "spinal stabilizer."

Herbal Therapies

Herbs are different from vitamins. They are derived from plants that are also used in the pharmaceutical industry. It is necessary that your doctor is aware of everything you are taking, even if it is not a prescription. While it may seem that herbs are harmless, there are situations where they could interfere with other medications. For some conditions, they are contraindicated. There can be variations in strength and quality among manufacturers, and for that reason, it is valuable to do your research on the company providing your herbs and supplements to ensure they are of excellent quality.

Detrimental Substances

Some other elements that affect patients may include both simple and complex issues, such as excessive coffee or alcohol intake. A patient may also have a slower response to care due to poor nutrition. It is well understood that both smoking and excessive alcohol consumption are detrimental to our health. Nicotine is a powerful drug that leeches minerals such as calcium from bone and decreases blood supply.

Alcohol should never be used as a means of self-medicating for chronic pain. Alcohol may act as a short-term muscle relaxant but provides no therapeutic effect and can adversely affect health and limit healing. Over time, other health problems may develop, such as high blood pressure, along with liver and digestive problems. Alcohol is a depressant, and those who abuse it can develop both physical and emotional dependency.

Physical Activity

When it comes to good health, movement is life. Staying fit is very important for our bodies, and this is especially true about the spine. It is important to maintain flexibility and range of motion, especially to heal after an injury or to decrease the effects of a degenerative disease.

One of the simplest and best ways to exercise is to walk. Walking strengthens the spine and maintains good overall health. I frequently recommend that patients lift some light weights to create resistance and rebuild muscles that may have atrophied from lack of use during an injury. You do not have to purchase expensive weights.

Exercise bands or even cans of vegetables provide enough resistance to help the spine. Stretching is very important as the muscles tend to spasm, which causes decreased blood flow. Stretching lengthens these muscles again, facilitating blood flow and increased oxygen levels.

Patients ask if they should focus on low-impact or high-impact exercise to get back into shape after a disc-related problem. The best avenue is to begin slowly. One of the biggest mistakes is to attempt to return to the level of exercise before the injury. When returning to exercise, it must begin slowly and moderately to avoid re-injury. Consistent exercise and gradually working up to the level of exercise previously enjoyed is important.

I had a patient in his early 40s, who was responding well to the DRS Protocol™, and he had achieved an 80% sustained improvement, after just a few weeks of care. Suddenly, he stopped making progress and even took a step back in improvement. We talked several times about what might be the problem.

After an additional two weeks of treatment and re-evaluation, he finally confessed he had started running again. His goal was to run in a race that was a month away. I strongly advised him to allow his spine to heal first, but he refused. Because he refused to comply with his treatment plan, I had to release him from care.

The patient was not able to complete the race, and he ended up having a spinal fusion. He did not run that year or any time thereafter, due to complications from his spinal fusion. This story illustrates that patience and focus are required to heal fully. The good from treatment can be undone, if the body is not allowed sufficient time to recover.

Early in the treatment with the DRS Protocol™, specific exercises such as running and weightlifting must be avoided, although this does not mean that the patient will never be able to resume these activities. It is important to avoid certain exercises that increase the disc pressure and cause re-injury of the disc.

One area of concern is exercise equipment. There is a variety of equipment including stationary bicycles, stair climbers, treadmills, and elliptical trainers. Riding a recumbent bicycle is great exercise when a patient is ready. However, equipment such as ellipticals may put unnatural stress on the spine and exacerbate a condition.

I approve the use of ellipticals only if the patient sets the equipment for little or no resistance. It is better to choose exercise equipment that will not alter the normal gait or biomechanics.

The benefits of exercising in the water are many. Aquatic exercise, such as swimming, improves cardiovascular fitness, endurance, and overall strength. Aquatic exercise gives the benefit of a non-weight bearing environment and reduces the likelihood of injury. Exercise balls are also popular and can help with balance and increasing the strength of core abdominal muscles. While using exercise balls is not for everyone, they are good for some patients. Simply balancing in a sitting position each day can help greatly. I use exercise balls in my practice because I have seen a great benefit for my patients who have used them to strengthen core muscles.

Every patient is different, so I recommend various stretches and exercises according to the needs and recovery of each. Once recovered, I encourage my patients to exercise regularly to keep their bodies in optimal shape to avoid another injury.

I also instruct my patients to continue the specific back or neck exercises they were given during the course of their treatment.

Dr. Richard Busch III

CHAPTER 9
Healing Starts in the Mind

CHAPTER 9
Healing Starts in the Mind

When I was in chiropractic college, professors would often discuss the philosophy of treating the whole person and not just the physical body. The role of the mind in healthcare has been observed for years, and there are competing schools of thought that are complex and multifaceted. There is a mind-body-spirit connection that is real and powerful. I know when I enlist my patients' minds in their own care, they respond faster.

We have all heard of people who were living normal, seemingly healthy lives, and suddenly they were diagnosed with a serious disease. Within a short time, some patients succumb to their diagnosis.

The fascinating psychological aspect of this is that what happens next may depend upon that person's perspective of the disease and the individual's beliefs. I believe the diagnosis, in many cases, can be as terminal as the disease.

When a patient is overcome with fear of the disease, and the fear has become thought, then the disease process is given the full strength and beliefs of the mind. This affects the body, and the thought is allowed to flourish. For some, this almost acts as a death sentence.

On the positive side, studies show that cancer patients who have positive attitudes toward the treatment and outcome of their disease have higher survival rates. Evidence suggests that what matters is the attitude toward the journey of treating the disease. This shows there are benefits to adopting a survivor attitude.

There are surgeons who will not operate on a patient if that patient is too mentally depressed or is convinced that the outcome will be less than favorable. When dealing with the human body, it is important to remember that it is not "just a body." There is also a "being", and the "being" brings its own memories, thoughts, and beliefs. These will affect the way that "being" responds to any type of care for any type problem.

The whole idea of a mind-body connection is that the attitude of the patient has a positive effect on a patient's overall health, recovery, and outcome. Guided imagery is used to work with and through this mind-body connection to aid in the healing process. Emotions can influence the immune system in either a positive or a negative way, and patients have the ability to choose, merely by their attitude.

It is important to understand the emotional, psychological, and mental factors that play into the healing of the patient. When I am dealing with a patient, I take all of this into consideration. It is much easier to help a patient who believes health is possible. Conversely, it is much harder to help someone who does not believe help is possible or is convinced that the situation is hopeless.

An area I focus on when treating someone is to teach the patient to perform visualization exercises or guided imagery for healing. I believe if the patient can see it and believe it; it is more likely to happen. There is also the verse from Proverbs: "As a man thinketh so is he." I believe this is most accurate.

The connection between a patient's state of mind and the ability to heal cannot be ignored. The mind is very powerful, and it can alter the way the body functions. With visualization exercises, the patient is removing any barriers that may be present in the way of thoughts and beliefs. In essence, the whole patient is being treated, not just the physical malady.

It does not matter how great treatment is, if the mind is not convinced about potential improvement, then no treatment will produce optimal results. For this reason, it is essential to recruit the mind into the equation.

I ask patients to visualize their lives without pain. I ask them to think about what they want to do and where they want to go, and to imagine and visualize all those activities that will suddenly be easy again—things such as getting in and out of a vehicle, being able to work all day, going to the grocery store or to the mall, or preparing a meal. This is especially important if a patient has been in pain for an extended period, as the pain takes away all focus, and it is difficult for a patient to even imagine being without it.

I also ask patients to imagine their bodies repairing the injured area. We look at illustrations of healthy vertebrae and discs, and then ask that they imagine healing, the inflammation disappearing, and their nerves being relieved from pressure. Patients are to do this for a few moments each treatment and again at home. It is important for patients to understand that they must do these visualization exercises each day.

Professional sports teams, Olympic athletes, and NASA have used visualization for years. What the mind can see, the body can achieve, and this same idea can be applied to healing. I was introduced to the idea of visualization through sports as a child.

When I was a boy, my dad coached my Little League baseball team. Before each game, he would have us all sit on the bench and visualize hitting the baseball, running the bases, making great catches, and winning the game.

My dad often said that to be prepared to win the game, first, you must play through the entire game in your mind and see yourself winning. Then, you are prepared to play optimally on the field.

Those principles are not just limited to sports and performance on the field of play. Many professional athletes perform the visualization exercises while recovering from an injury in an effort to speed the healing process.

While we are visualizing a certain activity, the brain does not recognize the difference between imagination and reality. As a result, the same area of the brain that receives input during an actual event is also firing and receiving input during the visualization exercises. This is important because as those centers of the brain fire, they cause the nerves to the muscles to fire, which speeds the healing process.

The mind-body connection is a growing area of interest in healthcare. After years of focusing completely on testing, prescription medication, and surgical procedures, the broader medical community is realizing that a patient's mindset has a direct correlation to the treatment outcome.

Some of the early tests revealed the "healing power" of the mind. These were double-blind studies performed where some of the test subjects were given real medications, and some were given placebos. High numbers of the subjects given placebos had improved results. Their improvement was attributed to their belief in what they were given, and that it could heal them.

These studies coined the phrase "placebo effect." Obviously, there is something much more important going on in healing—it is expectation and the power of the mind. Treating the complete person is an effective adjunct to any treatment. Patient mind power is something I have used for years in treating all my patients, and I have seen that they respond more quickly and have better results.

Occasionally, I have a patient who is resistant to the idea of visualization. I treated a patient named Mary Ann. She was a middle-aged woman who had injured her back moving some large potted plants in her home. I did a complete examination, and as I asked questions about her medical history, I noticed that she was relating extremely negative aspects of her life and her health.

She communicated that her life was awful and no one understood how she felt or sympathized with her condition. She also said that no one wanted to help her with anything. She blamed family, friends, other doctors, and anyone else she could think of for her problems.

Mary Ann was resistant to the idea of visualization. She could not imagine life without pain or struggle. She actively chose to view every person and event in her life in a negative way. Initially, I had limited improvement with Mary Ann, and she was pessimistic about the improvement she did experience.

Again, I sat down with her and discussed the importance of a positive attitude and the power of the visualization exercises. Mary Ann finally admitted to me that she was not following the recommendations and was not performing the exercises because she felt "stupid" doing them, and she did not continue them. After explaining the importance of the exercises for both her health and her life, she finally agreed to begin again.

From that point forward her health improved, as did her attitude toward life. These improvements were dramatic steps forward, and I am happy to report that her life changed in more than just physical improvement—this also helped improve her quality of life and the quality of her relationships. She had become a much happier and a more delightful person. It took a change in the way she viewed both her condition and her world to make a change, but the change was palpable.

As strange as it sounds, some of the patients I treat may have an emotional attachment to their pain. It is as if they do not want to let it go. The pain is one thing they have grown to count on and known as a constant. It becomes their purpose to discuss their condition with anyone who will listen. Everyone in the family becomes part of the suffering. This could be the natural part of the pain experience for some, but for others, health maladies may be an emotional crutch that excuses them from actively participating in life.

Other patients refuse to talk about their suffering with anyone. Perhaps, some feel there is no point in talking, as no one will understand anyway. Because pain is both a physical and psychological experience, there is a range of responses to pain. Patients who do not talk about their problems are the patients who may feel isolated and even shameful for not being able to buck up. They need visualization exercises the most, because if they cannot see recovery in their minds, they may continue to be disconnected, even from themselves, and never achieve it in their lives because negative emotions can rob and invalidate positive emotions.

Supportive Studies

More studies supporting the link between the mind and the body are presented every day. A study from the UCLA School of Medicine reported that stress and negative emotions have a physical impact on the immune system.[1] The protective end caps of cells, known as telomeres, remain long in those who have a positive outlook and less stress. Telomeres are indicators of the cell's ability to heal, and they show a direct link to our ability to stay well.

Another clinical study reported that subjects, all of whom had conditions that produced low white blood cell count including patients with cancer, AIDS, and other autoimmune deficiencies, used visualization and relaxation techniques each day, and after 90 days, all the subjects showed significant improvement in white blood cell counts.[2] There is a direct correlation between what we think and our body's healing abilities.

Expectation

When I am discussing treatment expectations with patients, I need to be certain we are both talking about the same thing. The expectations of patients are an important part of their care, and I address this immediately.

As an example, I explain to the patients who have had a back or neck problem for years that I am not going to be able to return their spine to that of a 20-year old, because there is a more significant degeneration now than when they were twenty. I need to know where the patient's mind is and what the starting perspective is. As the treatment progresses and pain diminishes, some patients forget how badly they felt before, and thus their expectations may rise to unrealistic levels.

I had such a conversation with a patient. She was in her mid-seventies, and I had treated her for many years. Her back pain had long been resolved. Occasionally, I treated her for supportive care. She told me she was upset because she was limited in what she was able to do. After a long discussion about this "problem," I pointed out that her frustration was about attempting activities that people half her age have trouble doing.

One of my favorite stories of a patient who experienced the opposite life change was Ruby, a 63-year-old grandmother. Ruby had become very comfortable in her life. Her routine included gardening, having the grandkids over every Sunday, and meeting her friend for lunch on occasion. She did not socialize much or go anywhere outside her set routines. That particular winter we had an extended ice storm, and Ruby had slipped on her porch and injured her lower back. Ruby's injury made her almost housebound. When I first met with Ruby, she told me that she felt she had aged twenty years and was afraid her back injury would be permanent. I had Ruby start on positive visualizations immediately, and she quickly responded to treatment.

It was not long before she was traveling abroad and taking cruises. Her injury and her recovery had highlighted to her that her good health is to be treasured and enjoyed. She was bubbly and positive, and this attitude had the effect of making her seem much younger than her 63 years. Many times, life gives what we expect to get. The same can be applied when recovering from an injury or dealing with a degenerative disease.

Another patient, named Jarrod, who had severe degeneration in the lumbar spine and was in his mid-fifties the first time I met with him. He brought an MRI for me to review. I have to admit that his MRI made me do a double take. The degeneration I saw in his spine was severe, and he had bone spurring off the front and back of the vertebrae. Jarrod also had a curve in his spine (scoliosis) that caused muscle spasms and chronic pain as well. The scoliotic curve may have been the cause of the degeneration. He was adamant that he did not want surgery.

I agreed to do what I could, although this was such a serious condition there could have been limitations to the care. Jarrod had been a builder his entire life, and he refused to let his condition slow him down. He used this same determination and responded very well to treatment. During the course of his care, Jarrod began developing an entire housing development, and he amazed me with his positive attitude.

I see many patients with ongoing degeneration in their spines that is caused by osteoarthritis, and I see others with damage to nerves, such as diabetic neuropathy. It is paramount for patients to understand that they may have a problem that is entirely unrelated to their disc condition, or, they may have a degenerative hip-related condition that is causing some of their pain.

When I see patients with unrelated conditions, I discuss their treatment alternatives, and I note that they have complicating factors that will not respond to the DRS Protocol™. It is essential for patients to understand they might have more than one condition that is playing a role in their symptoms. However, patients who have complicating factors can still achieve outstanding results for a disc-related condition with the DRS Protocol™.

The United States ranks number one in the use of surgery to treat back and neck pain. However, there are practitioners, including medical facilities, who offer nonsurgical spinal decompression which an integral part of the DRS Protocol™. However, not all offer the complete DRS Protocol™ that I have developed.

Many doctors simply treat with a spinal decompression table and offer a fixed number of treatments for a particular diagnosis. They are treating the diagnosis with a cookie-cutter approach, and they are not considering the overall patient. The DRS Protocol™ is customized for each patient and the specific condition. Each office is different and offers a different treatment program, and unless doctors have been trained by me, they do not offer the DRS Protocol™. As a side note: more and more doctors are being trained in the DRS Protocol™, so it is possible you may have a doctor in your area that has been trained. It is worth investigating.

A Positive Experience for Patients

Expectation is very important to create a positive experience with your doctor, and my office offers the DRS Protocol™. The DRS Protocol™ is patient-centered healthcare and focuses on the complete patient, not just a symptom or area of disease. With this approach, I am able to determine and customize the best treatment options for each patient to ensure my office provides the gold standard of care and keeps its main focus on the patient. My goal is to have my patients' healthcare experiences be as positive, easy, and comfortable as possible.

I explain from the beginning that the patient will be an active participant in care and not just an observer. This can be a very different relationship from what some patients may have experienced in other healthcare offices.

It is not uncommon for patients to be ignored or pushed out of their own healthcare decision-making process. Patients can become disillusioned by the lack of answers, attention, and compassion, as well as the great deal of time that must be invested by sitting in a doctor's waiting room. They may feel like a number.

The experience for the patient through the course of the DRS Protocol™ is a very comforting one. When treating for a low back problem, patients begin care by being placed on a spinal decompression table lying on their backs with a harness system placed around the pelvis and the thoracic spine or rib cage. As a computerized distractive force is applied via the pelvic harness, the patient will feel a gentle pulling sensation in and about the lumbar spine. Treatment is directed to the patient's particular disc level of injury by adjusting the angle of force. The force is applied from a specific angle that is dependent upon the disc level being treated, and this varies from patient to patient. The amount of force to be applied is customized to each patient's individual condition and weight.

When treating the cervical spine, the amount of distractive force is again formulated based on the patient's condition and size and will be significantly less than the distractive force for the lumbar spine. Cervical patients are also placed on a decompression table lying on their back. The patient's head and neck are stabilized in a cradle that extends around the back of the skull, or the occiput, and a very gentle distractive force is applied to the specified disc level.

After finishing with the spinal decompression portion of care, the patient then undergoes separate physical therapy modalities, such as electrical stimulation, ultrasound, low level laser, ice/heat, and others (depending on what that particular patient's needs are), to reduce inflammation further while allowing the body to release its own natural painkillers and allowing the body to heal.

The goal is stabilization and pain relief, which is not only the result of the disc healing, but also the result of exercise and nutrition used in conjunction with the rest of the treatment to help rebuild and strengthen the body.

During a short beginning phase of care, patients are treated on a daily basis. Thereafter, the frequency decreases dependent upon their progress. My mindset, about treatment and everything I do in my office, is to look at each patient as an individual and base care on the individual's situation.

There are many elements of the protocol. The DRS Protocol™ is not just a treatment using a particular type of spinal decompression table or therapies; it includes the positive experiences for a patient—from the first telephone call to my office to the complete course of the patient's care. All elements are involved in the success of the care.

I have treated many patients who were previously treated by another doctor with spinal decompression without having achieved the best results. When patients receive treatment with the DRS Protocol™, they quickly realize that their care is much more involved. Their response to care is a positive outcome.

CHAPTER 10
A Life Without Pain

CHAPTER 10
A Life Without Pain

When someone is suffering from back or neck pain, there is no reason to be fearful of treatment and to continue living in pain. There is a successful and noninvasive alternative—the DRS Protocol™, even if you have tried physical therapy, injections, and even surgery.

My purpose in writing *Surgery not Included* is to inform both patients and healthcare providers of the successful, nonsurgical option of the DRS Protocol™. This information is intended to inform those suffering from chronic pain that surgery is not their only option. Their treatment path does not need to be long, frustrating, and full of mediocre results.

One such case was Gavin. When I first examined Gavin, he was skeptical, angry, and having severe back pain. He had been to several doctors and two surgeons. Each one told him he absolutely had to have surgery. By the time he came to me, he was not sleeping due to his discomfort, and he was short-tempered and borderline abusive. He was what I would call "very difficult."

Pain, anger, and fear can go hand-in-hand. When a chronic pain patient is told there is only one frightening solution—and it is not a good solution—frustration can boil over. Some take it out on everyone around them, including those who are trying to help.

It took a great deal of patience to get through Gavin's evaluation. He even tested the patience of my staff, and they have been

Dr. Richard Busch III

trained to work with patients who are in pain. It is sad to say how common this is, but I treat a high percentage of patients who have severe and chronic disc conditions, and they are suffering.

Gavin had lived with pain for years. He had degenerative disc disease in his lower back, and he recently had fallen and exacerbated his back problem. He was experiencing shooting pain down both legs. I reviewed my exam and X-ray findings with him and discussed treatment with the DRS Protocol™. Based on his experiences with doctors, he was more than reluctant.

Nevertheless, he did not want surgery, so he said, "I'll try", all the while telling me he thought all "blanking" doctors were quacks. We talked about his attitude of implied failure. I told Gavin that "just trying" was not a strong enough commitment to produce the best outcome. He agreed, and we moved forward.

Within the first few treatments with the DRS Protocol™, the pain in both legs had significantly decreased, and Gavin was definitely getting around much better. After a few weeks, he seemed like a new man. He was finally sleeping and being rested brightened his whole outlook. While it did not completely change his personality, it did improve his demeanor a great deal.

Loved Ones

Family members of patients can sometimes help, and they can sometimes hurt. They can be so fed up with their loved one's complaints that they demand they come to see me. On the other hand, they can also be so convinced that surgery is the only way, that they discourage their loved ones from being assessed for the DRS Protocol™.

In other cases, the family might discount altogether the patient's problem by inferring, "It's all in your head." Or, for a number of reasons, they may actually interfere with the patient's decision-making.

Margie was such a patient. One of her dearest friends is also a patient of mine, and she strongly encouraged Margie to see me.

It was winter, and she had a misstep off a curb, slipping on the ice. The result for Margie was a herniated disc accompanied by severe back and leg pain.

A close family member of Margie's was working for a surgeon and tried to convince her that treating with the DRS Protocol™ or with chiropractic care might cause severe damage or even stroke. Scientific studies clearly indicate that there is no significant risk for stroke from chiropractic care, and chiropractic treatment is safer than most medical treatments.[1] DRS Protocol™ has no negative side effects. Sometimes other conditions, such as symptoms of what was assumed to be diabetic neuropathy, elevated blood pressure due to pain and stress, or incontinence, may clear up when the pressure on the nerves is removed.

Thankfully, Margie agreed to treatment, and within a few weeks, she made a full recovery with more than 95% improvement. Later, Margie's close family member became a patient of mine.

The Simple Truth

I focus on providing a thorough layman's explanation to be certain my patients clearly understand the diagnosis and course of treatment. It is also important for patients to be able to explain their diagnosis and treatment to others.

One of my first lessons in this, as a young doctor, occurred a number of years ago, when a woman named Ollie May came to see me. At the time, she was in her mid-to-late seventies and was a very sweet and delightful person. While examining her X-rays, I noticed that she had an abdominal aortic aneurysm (a section where the artery balloons out). She had neglected to mention this in her medical history.

Many times, patients do not understand why they need to tell a chiropractor about all health conditions and concerns. I asked her about the aneurysm, and she said she was aware of it and so was her cardiologist.

As I always do when patients have serious complicating conditions, I planned to contact Ollie May's cardiologist, later that day, to discuss her treatment plan, confirming it would not interfere with any other treatment or problem with her aneurysm. When working with patients with ongoing disease processes such as heart disease, diabetes, aneurysms, transplants, and others, I look very closely at the treatment they are receiving for conditions outside of my care.

When appropriate, I get clearance from their other physicians prior to beginning treatment. I send a complete report to the patient's specialists, so they are fully aware of the treatment I will be providing to a patient. This assures the patient that there is an adequate exchange of information about medical history and that the treatment will be performed with the knowledge of everyone involved in care.

I knew I could help Ollie May with the pain she was experiencing in her back and legs. She left my office quite happy with this knowledge, but before my office could contact her cardiologist, I received a call from him. The conversation started with, "What exactly are you doing over there?"

Apparently, I had said something that Ollie May had interpreted somehow as my saying I could treat her aneurysm in addition to her disc. I had told her that I could treat her back condition despite the aneurysm. Ollie May had called her cardiologist and told him that I was going to treat her leg and back pain as well as fix her aneurysm, which was not the case. After a short explanation, the cardiologist approved treatment with the DRS Protocol™, and we had a good chuckle. However, I never forgot the lesson that if you do not explain things clearly and thoroughly, patients may fill in the blanks with the wrong information.

Never assume anything anyone repeats is 100% accurate— whether it is good or bad. Very often, patients come to my office for care after being seen by another doctor, and they tell me their back pain is the result of one leg being shorter than the other leg. In many cases, this is not the cause of the pain; it is a symptom of a biomechanical alteration and may not be permanent. Each patient's experience, medical history, and current medical condition are unique. There are no absolutes or across-the-board treatments when dealing with back and neck pain. Each situation must be evaluated by a qualified professional. Do not let someone else's opinion discourage you. Opinions and procedures may vary from city to city and region to region. There are alternatives available.

You are in Charge

Many patients believe that they do not have control over their healthcare—but they do. It is true that insurance companies often dictate care. It is also true that patients are conditioned to simply go along with doctors' recommendations. Therefore, they do not seek other treatment options. Some doctors are used to patients going along with recommendations without question. When a patient does ask questions, some doctors may become irritated because they are just not used to questions.

A doctor should not forget that patients know their bodies and how they feel—doctors do not know everything about each specific patient, so just listening to a patient is critical.

I frequently treat patients with chronic pain who have been told by a doctor, at some point in their search for help, that perhaps stress or a relationship problem is the culprit, and perhaps there really is not a physical problem. This infers (if the doctor has not stated it outright) that "it is all in their head."

When the doctor, an authority figure, questions a person's reality, it can convince a patient that it is just destiny, and they have to live with pain and suffering. This is humiliating and stops some patients from investigating options because they are afraid they will experience the same embarrassing assumption again. Or they are told to try a new medication and, "let's see what happens." This may be construed as a brush-off. It is discouraging and again causes patients to question themselves.

How many times have you watched a commercial about a prescription drug, one with a long, rapidly-read list of possible side effects and have wondered who in their right mind would ever take that drug? The side effects are often worse than the condition the drugs are intended to cure. When a patient wants a doctor to provide a simple and fast solution, the doctor's decision is often affected by pharmaceutical sponsored advertising.

Patients take some of the most harmful drugs because they believe they are needed since a doctor prescribed them and perhaps because their insurance covers the drugs. Yet the entire list of the potential side effects may have never been fully explained, so some side effects come as a complete shock to the patient. I treat many patients who are taking so many medications that it is difficult to differentiate their true medical issues from drug-related side effects or drug interactions. A well-known example is statins, which are prescribed for lowering cholesterol. Some doctors estimate that 15% of patients taking statins are affected in some manner. A prevalent symptom is mild to severe muscle cramping and spasms, and of a higher concern are elevated liver enzymes. Frequently, I treat patients who have had to discontinue their cholesterol medications, and miraculously their leg pain goes away.

There are also central nervous system complaints from statins which translate as cognitive (memory) problems, although up until recently, side effects like fuzzy thinking and loss of memory were not listed on the drug information sheets.

However, some doctors had noticed changes like these: Dr. Orli Etinging, Vice Chair of Medicine of New York Presbyterian Hospital, stated in the *Wall Street Journal* article, "Do Statins Make You Stupid?", February 12, 2008, that she had witnessed cognitive deficits (in women) that were on statins. When the drugs were discontinued - the problems discontinued. There are also reports of irritability, aggression, and personality changes. These types of changes and problems are difficult to test and gauge and are easy for doctors to dismiss.

The brain is an organ and is 2.3 percent of the body's total weight, yet is made of 25 percent of the total cholesterol in the body. Cholesterol plays a primary role in the operation of the brain: cholesterol is in every cell of the body. However, the cholesterol in the brain is distinctive and separate from the cholesterol in the rest of the body. Then, the question is, would it be probable that people who take a cholesterol-lowering drug be affected by diminished learning and memory?

It is difficult to draw firm conclusions because studies haven't focused heavily on this particular point. However, there are smaller studies and reports such as the study, "Better memory functioning associated with higher total and low-density lipoprotein cholesterol levels in very elderly subjects without the apolipoprotein e4 allele", *Am J Geriatr Psychiatry*, 2008, Sep16.[2]

This study determined that of the "oldest old people" are those who have the highest cholesterol levels, and surprisingly they have better memories. The brain must have cholesterol to function.

From my observations over the years, I am seeing an elevated number of patients who are on statin drugs. This is not surprising, because the acceptable numbers for cholesterol levels have been lowered, therefore most doctors are encouraging patients to reach the newest recommended numbers and are following the newest medical guidelines. Along with increased statin-takers, I am also seeing more people who are exhibiting signs of dementia.

I recently consulted with a patient who was taking statins . She immediately stated she had a high-level of memory loss and symptoms of dementia. After she had thoroughly discussed her memory problems with her prescribing doctor, they mutually agreed she should immediately stop taking her statin medication.

The result was, within three weeks, the patient regained normal levels of awareness. This is exactly what the FDA reports in the fine print warnings about statin side effects: *"Usually memory loss and forgetfulness, for most should return to normal within three weeks of discontinuing the drug."*

No one should instantly discontinue taking statins. If you feel you have symptoms of dementia and memory loss among others, discuss this with your prescribing doctor before making any changes. It is highly recommended, if possible, to work toward lifestyle changes and improved diet and exercise to naturally lower cholesterol. Patients and family members should do their own research.

I will never forget a patient named Ellen who came in with a list of medications so long that I honestly had to wonder if her doctors truly had her best interests at heart. She was taking many medications, and some were prescribed just to combat the side effects of other medications. Ellen was taking stroke medications, blood thinners, diuretics, drugs to sleep, drugs to wake up, pain medications, drugs for heart disease and cholesterol, drugs for blood pressure, two for diabetes, one for neuropathy, one for diarrhea, and one for acid reflux.

This is not to say that Ellen did not have health issues, but she never questioned the amount of medications or the types of medications that were prescribed. Every time she had a problem, she would go back to see her doctor or another specialist, and she would come back with another medication. In defense of her doctors, they were treating her conditions.

Doctors have to listen to their patients and pay attention to what they are being told. With the list of drugs Ellen was taking, one has to wonder if anyone was listening and how adding more drugs made sense. Even with the help of the Medicare or insurance prescription programs, there still have to be expenses involved in filling that many prescriptions,. There comes the point where the patient and the doctor must communicate.

My grandfather was told he had three months to live. He immediately stopped taking his medications since some had unpleasant side effects anyway. When my grandfather saw his doctor, he told the doctor that he had discontinued his medications. The doctor said that he needed to take, at least, the heart medications or he would die. My grandfather quickly replied, "You just told me I am going to die, and that stuff is expensive!"

The interesting point is my grandfather felt much better after discontinuing his medications. Yes, he did pass away, but nine months later. Obviously, patients should consult with their doctors before discontinuing any medications.

The lesson about Ellen is to ask questions. Even family members who notice their loved ones are being prescribed more and more medications should be proactive and ask some questions. The truth is that the body has tremendous abilities to heal without the long-term use of drugs.

The problem with many prescription drugs is that they stop vital reactions and processes of the body. When that happens, there cannot be normal health, and there have to be side effects. Certain medications and even drug interactions can slow the healing process.

Taking charge of your healthcare and committing to gain knowledge about your body and how to heal naturally will decrease the need for prescriptions and invasive procedures for disc-related conditions. My main goal in writing *Surgery not Included* is to provide the knowledge that many patients need to make informed healthcare decisions.

Patients frequently come to my office and tell me what treatments their previous doctors have recommended. However, they rarely can tell me what their diagnosis was or what it meant. It is important to know exactly what is to be treated, and why, before agreeing to a procedure. Many times, the problem is simply with communication.

Doctors do not always communicate effectively, if at all. Remember that the medical system does not allow much time for listening and eliciting information from patients, and patients do not always report properly and are afraid to ask questions. This alone can lead to unnecessary suffering. I take time to educate my patients, so they know exactly what is wrong, that way they can take an active role in their own care.

Every person is unique and needs to be treated as such. Just because some doctors treat patients like numbers does not mean we should accept it.

The body is a wonderfully created machine and, if allowed, most disc conditions can heal more perfectly, given the proper environment, than anything done with invasive treatment can achieve. This is the philosophy of chiropractic care and the DRS Protocol™ with spinal decompression. I teach this protocol to doctors across the country. We can help patients without inflicting trauma.

My goal is to get the patient well. I have dedicated my life to helping sick and suffering people. Through the years, I have had many employees who were registered nurses. Some had extensive experience in different healthcare settings, from the hospital ER to the family doctor. Each one has said the same thing: "I love working here; the office is full of happy people, and they get well!"

Your Choices Matter

More than 90% of overall health is due to lifestyle and environmental factors that influence our health. This means that most adults have an extraordinary amount of control over their health through the choices made every day. This includes everything from avoiding those items that we know are detrimental, as well as following a balanced diet, and getting some form of exercise. There is much misinformation about what the body needs, what constitutes a healthy lifestyle, and what qualifies as a balanced diet. Double check your sources.

In general terms, you cannot go wrong when buying organic meats, fruits, and vegetables, and staying away from processed foods. This is because nonorganic foods are treated with substances that are harmful to the body or mimic hormones within the body, and those can cause disease. The higher the quality of food you put into your body, the better you will feel and the fewer problems you will have.

On occasion, when I mention this, I get the standard response from patients that organic is expensive and just too much trouble, although now organic products are readily available in most grocery stores.

Yet, when the cost of organic foods is compared to the cost of prescription drugs and medical procedures to treat the disease processes caused by pesticides, hormones, and other negative, external influences—then organic foods could be considered a bargain.

Smoking is detrimental to healing. Some studies indicate that there are over 2,000 chemicals in cigarette smoke, and these all cause problems with the way your body functions. Not only does smoking shorten your life span, it also severely inhibits your ability to recover from an injury.

Smokers rarely achieve the best treatment outcomes. That is sad and unnecessary, which is why I discourage my patients' smoking. Even if I am able to discourage my patients from smoking for only the duration of their treatment, they will have a greater advantage to achieve maximum healing.

The discontinuation of destructive habits, such as smoking or drinking alcohol excessively, coupled with encouraging positive aspects, like exercise and eating an organic diet, will have tremendous, positive long-term effects.

One of the best actions anyone can take to improve health is to stop destructive or harmful habits. Working with our natural processes and paying attention when our body tells us something is wrong is also one of the best preventive strategies.

A frequent situation I encounter is patients who have allowed their pain condition to go on for years, and therefore, the wait may have caused unnecessary damage. By listening to your body and getting help early, rather than waiting, you can have positive results.

One of my patients, named Jerry, worked as a truck driver for over 20 years. He was overweight, and the stress and strain of his job had resulted in on-and-off lower back pain. He had been suffering from back problems for more than ten years.

He popped ibuprofen as if it were candy, and he frequently slept sitting in a recliner, because his legs became numb when he was lying down. Jerry did not feel the need to see a doctor about these problems until he reached a point that his pain was interfering with his ability to work.

This is very common, especially with men, and particularly if their pain has not been debilitating. They adjust to higher levels of pain, and if it does not keep them from working, they do not think it is bad enough to visit the doctor. Jerry was just this type of guy.

I see this often with farmers, construction workers, and truck drivers. All of them, and there are certainly others, are hardworking, do not offer excuses, and have a strong work ethic. Yet, this is bad because the body is saying, "something is wrong."

The body is trying to protect the spinal structure. Delaying means increased swelling, more nerve damage, and more deterioration. Some of these changes will be permanent if not corrected in time.

Jerry was treated with the DRS Protocol™ and had an excellent outcome with more than 90% improvement. He recognized that correcting smaller back problems early would prevent debilitating ones later. It is this realization that causes many patients to refer their family members and friends for care. They understand that more severe problems are created by waiting.

Focus on the "After"

We have all seen the advertising of the before-and-after photos of people who have had tremendous weight loss. I often wish I had something similar to show the dramatic changes we create in people's lives by helping their pain. Even though they appear the same on the outside, their attitudes and outlooks on life have changed.

For those who are currently in pain and wondering if the DRS Protocol™ with spinal decompression may offer the answer, I would encourage them to focus on the "after." Much like the visualization exercises I give patients to perform, and that is believing that he or she can get well and believing that there is a nonsurgical solution as the first step to living a full and pain-free life.

I often find that patients in pain resign themselves to their lives. They do not look ahead or think about tomorrow. Because they are in pain, they can focus only on today and getting through it. Before long, their lives turn inward and become a daily grind of pain upon more pain. Usually, after a few days of treatment with the DRS Protocol™, they begin to see beyond today and then look forward to tomorrow. Before long, they are reviving lost dreams.

Because I have taught this protocol to other doctors, patients have more and more access to effective and safe alternatives that can give them back the lives they once had. I always ask my patients to rate their percentage of improvement. This is a way to compare their pain reduction, as opposed to their pain level when they started care. Rating their improvement allows them to realize the vast amount of progress they have made in a very short time.

While I always emphasize that if you are 50 years old, you will not physically return to the way you were when you were 20, but you also will not feel as if you are 75 or 80. The goal is to get the patient to feel as well as possible for the given age and state of health. In that respect, I have seen tremendous success.

Your Partner in Healthcare

Within the pages of this book, I have conveyed not only my medical knowledge and expertise but also my philosophy about patient care. I feel strongly that I am a partner with my patients on their journey to recovery. I am not a commander but a coach, an expert with the tools to help them to complete the process of becoming free from pain.

An important aspect of all care I provide including the DRS Protocol™ is that the patient is treated as a special human being. We all have wants, needs, and desires, and we consist of more than our physical bodies. When doctors ignore the emotional and spiritual aspects of what it is to be human, they shortchange the patient's overall health and only treat a symptom.

I believe the foundation of patient care is in the relationship between the doctor and patient, one that we build together. I have a strong commitment to seeing my patients through their care and to a positive outcome. I want to assure anyone who is suffering from back or neck pain or peripheral neuropathy that there is hope. We have always known the body can heal itself, if give the proper situation, and that is what we are doing.

You do not have to live in pain or debilitation. Do not wait one more day to begin your new life, living free of pain and full of the promise of a bright and active future. *Surgery not Included.*

GLOSSARY

Acute pain: Resulting from a specific incident of tissue damage as in, burning a finger on a hot iron.

Alkaline phosphatase: An enzyme originating from the liver, bone, or the placenta. This is released into the blood when an injury occurs and during bone growth.

Allopathic doctors: Medical doctors who use methods of treating disease by the use of agents that produce effects different from those the disease treated.

Amputee: Individual who has lost one or both legs due to trauma or disease.

Amitriptyline: A medication used to treat various forms of depression, pain associated with the nerves (neuropathic pain), and to prevent migraine headaches. It is sold in the United States under the brand names Elavil® and Endep® and also helps patients sleep.

Anatomy: The study of form. Gross anatomy involves structures that can be seen with the naked eye as opposed to microscopic anatomy (or histology) which involves structures seen under the microscope. Traditionally, both gross and microscopic anatomy have been studied in the first year of medical school in the U.S. The most celebrated textbook of anatomy in the English-speaking world is Gray's Anatomy, still a useful reference book.

Aneurysm: An area of an artery, vein, or the heart that has weakened and is bulging or threatening to rupture.

Ankylosing spondylitis: A type of arthritis that causes chronic inflammation of the spine and the sacroiliac joints. This can lead

Dr. Richard Busch III

to pain and stiffness in the spinal region. This condition can lead to a natural fusion of the vertebrae causing total loss of motion in the spinal region.

Arachnoiditis: A debilitating condition characterized by severe stinging, burning pain, and neurologic problems.

Arthritis: Inflammation of a joint. There are well over 100 types of arthritis, which can leave the joints inflamed resulting in stiffness, swelling, and pain.

Articular cartilage: Cartilage that covers the articular surfaces of bones.

Artificial disc: An artificial disc is a device that is surgically implanted into the spine to replace the natural disc, and imitate the functions of a normal disc.

Aspirin: The common name for acetylsalicylic acid. Patients often use this as their first line of pain relief.

Atherosclerosis: Progressive thickening and hardening of the walls of arteries as a result of fat deposits.

Bacteria: Single-celled microorganisms, which can exist either as independent organisms or as parasites. Bacterial infections can range from mild to life threatening. Infection is a common surgical complication.

Biological barrier: A biological barrier forms when the cut that forms the scar tissue is made with a sharp object (such as a scalpel) leaving an impenetrable wall that will not heal properly over time. To understand this further, we can compare it to transplanting a plant to a large pot. If you try to replant the plant in a larger pot without first roughening up the root ends (from a clean cut), the roots will not take because in essence they have created a biological barrier.

Blood: Fluid in the body that transports all the elements necessary for life including water, nutrient, minerals and oxygen.

The discs between the vertebrae absorb these essential items through a process called diffusion.

Blood pressure: The pressure placed on the arterial wall by the blood as it circulates through the body. Elevated blood pressure is an indicator of possible heart disease or risk of stroke.

Bone: Bone is the hard substance that forms the skeleton of the human body. Its composition is mainly calcium phosphate and calcium carbonate. Bone also serves as a storage area for calcium, playing a large role in calcium balance in the blood.

Bowel: Another name for the intestine. The small bowel and the large bowel are the small intestine and large intestine and process all the food we take in. Some pain medications can cause gastrointestinal bleeds.

Brain: The part of the central nervous system that is located within the skull. The brain functions as the primary receiver, organizer and distributor of information for the body. Pain is received and processed in the brain and each person perceives pain differently.

Calcitonin: A hormone produced by the thyroid gland that lowers the levels of calcium and phosphate in the blood. This hormone promotes the formation of new bone.

Cannula: A tube inserted into a bodily cavity that may be used to administer a substance.

Cartilage: Tissue with a firm, rubbery consistency that cushions bones at joints. Tendons and ligaments are made of a more flexible type of cartilage and connect muscles with bones and make up other parts of the body, such as the larynx and the exterior of the ears.

CAM (Complementary and Alternative Medicine): Complementary and alternative medicine is a group of diverse medical and healthcare systems, practices, and products that are not generally considered part of conventional medicine.

CAT scan: The CAT (Computerized Axial Tomography) scan, also known as the CT (computed tomography) scan, is an X-ray technique that produces pictures representing a detailed cross section of body's tissue.

Chronic pain: Pain that has lasted beyond the 3-6 month time frame for tissue healing. This type of pain is ongoing and more constant than acute pain.

Complication: This is an additional problem that arises following a procedure, surgery or treatment. This can add to the difficulty of recovery for the patient or extend the recovery period.

Compression fracture: A hairline break in a bone cause by hitting another bone and being "compressed."

Cortisone: This is an adrenocorticoid hormone, a naturally occurring hormone made by and secreted by the adrenal cortex, the outer part of the adrenal gland. Cortisone is useful in reducing inflammation.

Cauda equina: A bundle of spinal nerve roots that arise from the bottom end of the spinal cord.

Cox 2 inhibitors: Drugs used to treat the pain and swelling of arthritis inflammation.

Dexa scan: Bone density scan that gives an actual risk score.

Degenerative arthritis: This is also known as osteoarthritis, this type of arthritis is caused by inflammation of cartilage in the joints and an eventual breakdown and loss of that cartilage. This is the most common type of arthritis.

Diabetes: A chronic disease characterized by high glucose levels within the body. Can cause diabetic neuropathy as the glucose levels make the nerves deteriorate.

Diagnosis: The identification of a particular disease or condition.

Glossary

Disc: In relation to the spine, this is an intervertebral disc, a disc-shaped piece of specialized tissue that separates the bones of the spine and prevents them rubbing against one another.

Discogram: A diagnostic test where the doctor injects dye into the disc. A very painful test that also destroys the disc.

Discectomy: Excision, in part or whole, of an intervertebral disc.

Dysesthesia: Impairment of sensitivity especially to touch.

Epidural space: The outermost part of the spinal canal.

Epidural injection: Medication delivered into the spinal cavity. For back pain, usually a mixture of anti-inflammatory and pain medication.

EMG (Electromyography): Involves testing the electrical activity of muscles. It is a test used to evaluate electrical impulses from the nerves.

ED (Erectile dysfunction): Is the inability of a man to maintain a firm erection long enough to have sex.

Estrogen: Estrogen is a female hormone produced by the ovaries. Phytoestrogens can cause undesirable effects and are found in soy products. Estrogen deficiency can lead to osteoporosis.

Extremity: These are used to refer to the hands and feet. Many patients have tingling or numbness in their extremities.

Examination: The doctor/patient time used for evaluating a person's physical condition and medical history.

Facet joints: Facet joints occur in pairs at the back of each vertebra. The facet joints link the vertebrae directly above and below to form a working unit that permits movement of the spine.

Foramina: A small opening in the bone through which nerves pass

Fracture: A break in bone or cartilage. Degenerative diseases and loss of calcium can make bones prone to fracture.

Functional scoliosis: A structurally normal spine that appears to have a lateral curve (scoliosis).

Herniated disc: Rupturing of the intervertebral disc tissue that separates the vertebral bones of the spinal column. The tissue herniates out of position and can press on the nerves of the spine.

Herniation: Abnormal extrusion of tissue through an opening. For example, an intervertebral disc located between vertebrae can push out of position and press against nerves.

Hormone: A chemical substance produced in the body that controls and regulates the activity of certain cells or organs.

Iliac: Pertaining to the ilium, the lowest part of the abdominal regions.

Incontinence: Urinary incontinence refers to the inability to keep urine in the bladder. Nerve compression sometimes causes incontinence problems.

Inflammation: An immune response to injury, irritation or infection. Inflammation causes swelling, redness and pain.

Injury: Trauma inflicted on the body inducing acute pain or damage to tissues.

Joint: The point where two bones come together and allow articulation of the body. Joints contain fibrous connective tissue and cartilage.

Laminectomy: A surgical procedure in which the posterior arch of a vertebra is removed. Laminectomy is done to relieve pressure on the spinal cord or on the nerve roots that emerge from the spinal canal. The procedure may be used to treat a slipped or herniated disc or to treat spinal stenosis.

Glossary

Ligament: A sheet or band of tough, fibrous tissue connecting bones or cartilages at a joint or supporting an organ.

Low back pain: Pain in the region known as the lower back can indicate problems with the lumbar spine, the discs between the vertebrae, the ligaments around the spine and discs, the spinal cord and nerves, muscles of the lower back, internal organs of the pelvis and abdomen, or the skin covering the lumbar area.

Lumbar radiculopathy: Nerve irritation caused by damage to the discs between the vertebrae. Damage to the disc occurs because of normal wear and tear of the outer ring of the disc, injury, or both. As a result, the gel-like center portion of the disc can herniate through the outer ring of the disc and press against the spinal cord or its nerves as they exit the bony spinal column. This can cause the commonly recognized pain known as sciatica that shoots down the leg.

Lumbar strain: A stretching injury to the ligaments, tendons, and/or muscles of the low back. The stretching incident results in microscopic tears of varying degrees in these tissues. Lumbar strain is one of the most common causes of low back pain. The injury can occur because of overuse, improper use, or trauma. It is classified as "acute" if it has been present for days to weeks. If the strain lasts longer than 3 months, it is referred to as "chronic."

Lumbar vertebrae: There are five lumbar vertebrae. These vertebrae are situated between the thoracic vertebrae and the sacral vertebrae in the spinal column. The five lumbar vertebrae are represented by the symbols L1 through L5.

Lymph fluid: An almost colorless fluid that travels through vessels called lymphatics in the lymphatic system and carries cells that help fight infection and disease.

MRI: Acronym for magnetic resonance imaging, which produces images of the soft tissues of the body by detecting differences in tissue density.

MRSA bacteria: Drug resistant strain of flesh eating bacteria known to thrive in many hospitals. This infection can be a complication of surgery.

Muscle: Muscle is the tissue of the body, which primarily creates movement. There are three types of muscle in the body. Muscle that is responsible for moving extremities and external areas of the body is called skeletal muscle. Heart muscle is called cardiac muscle. Muscle that is in the walls of arteries and bowel is called smooth muscle.

Muscle-guarding: Spasm of the muscles that occurs after a back or neck injury. A protection mechanism of the body.

Musculoskeletal: Relating to or involving the muscles and the skeleton.

Myelogram: An X-ray of the spinal cord after a contrast dye is injected.

Myelofibrosis: Fibrosis (spontaneous scarring) of the bone marrow.

NSAIDs (nonsteroidal anti-inflammatory drugs): These include aspirin, ibuprofen (Advil® and Motrin®), naproxen sodium (Aleve®), and ketoprofen (Orudis KT®).

Nerve: Fibers made up of trillions of individual nerve cells that transmit electrical impulses from the body to the brain for interpretation.

Nerve ablation: Destruction of the nerve through radio waves.

Nerve conduction velocity (NCV): Tests the electrical function of the nerve itself.

Nerve root: Nerve branching off from the spinal cord.

Neurological: Medical specialty concerned with treating the nervous system: Brain, spinal cord, and nerves.

Neuropathy: Pain along the path of a nerve.

Glossary

Off label drug use: The practice of prescribing pharmaceuticals for a purpose outside the scope of a drug's approved label.

Osteoarthritis: A type of arthritis caused by inflammation, breakdown, and eventual loss of cartilage in the joints.

Osteomyelitis: Inflammation of the bone due to infection. Osteomyelitis can be a complication of surgery or injury, although infection can also reach bone tissue through the bloodstream. Both the bone and the bone marrow may be infected. Symptoms include deep pain and muscle spasms in the area of inflammation, and fever.

Osteoporosis: Reduction in bone mass due to depletion of calcium and bone protein. Osteoporosis can make the bones fragile and prone to fractures, which are often slow to heal and heal poorly. It is more common in older adults, particularly post-menopausal women; in patients on steroids; and in those who take steroidal drugs. Unchecked osteoporosis can lead to changes in posture, physical abnormality and decreased mobility.

Orthopedic: Specialty involved in taking care of the skeletal system.

Pain: An unpleasant feeling that can range from mild, localized discomfort to agony. Pain has both physical and emotional components. The physical part of pain results from nerve stimulation. Pain is carried to the brain along nerve fibers for interpretation. Every person perceives pain differently.

Paraspinal Muscles: Muscles adjacent to the spine that support the movement of the spine.

Pelvis: The lower part of the abdomen located between the hip bones.

Percutaneous: Under the skin.

Phantom pain: The sensation that the injury is still present long after the site has healed. In amputees, the sensation that the limb is still there long after amputation.

216   *Dr. Richard Busch III*

Physical therapy: Rehabilitative healthcare that uses specially designed exercises and equipment to help patients regain or improve their physical abilities. Physical therapy is one of the first treatments given to back pain sufferers.

Photomodulation: Light therapy utilizing the correct frequency and wavelength of light that works as a result of the photoreceptors in the cells and organelles of cells. Affects cellular function and metabolism of the cells by stimulating the mitochondrial function to increase cellular energy and nitric oxide production for increased oxygenation of the cells and surrounding tissue.

Prostaglandins: One of a number of hormone-like substances that participate in a wide range of body functions.

Protein: A large molecule composed of one or more chains of amino acids in a specific order determined by the base sequence of nucleotides in the DNA coding for the protein.

Radiate: To start in one location and spread out. Pain may radiate from one point and affect several parts of the body.

Radiculopathy: Any disease of the spinal nerve roots and spinal nerves.

Rotation and flexion and extension: This refers to a range of motion.

Sacrum: Made up of fused sacral vertebrae, the sacrum is the large heavy bone located at the base of the spine. The sacrum is located in the spinal column, between the lumbar vertebrae and the coccyx. It is somewhat triangular in shape and is largely the back wall of the pelvis. The female sacrum is wider and less curved than the male to allow for childbirth.

Scar tissue: The fibrous tissue that the body creates to replace damaged skin is called a scar. Scars are also known as cicatrices and are formed as a biological response for repairing skin and other tissue damage in the human body

Glossary

Sciatica: Pain resulting from inflammation of or pressure on, the sciatic nerve. This type of pain is typically felt from the lower back to under the buttocks, radiating down below the knee. Sciatica frequently results from a herniated disc directly pressing on the nerve, but can because by any irritation or inflammation.

Scoliosis: Lateral curvature of the spine.

Somatovisceral referred pain: The combination of nerve pain from organs, skin and musculoskeletal origins.

Spasm: Involuntary repeated awkward jerking movements. A muscle spasm cause tremendous pain as the muscles contract. Nerve pain in the spine can cause the surrounding muscles to spasm.

Spinal cord: The main bundle of nerve tissue that is connected to the brain and lies within the vertebral canal. Thirty-one pairs of spinal nerves originate in the spinal cord: 8 cervical, 12 thoracic, 5 lumbar, 5 sacral, and 1 coccygeal. The spinal cord and the brain make up the central nervous system. The spinal cord consists of nerve fibers that transmit impulses to and from the brain.

Spinal fluid: Fluid located within the spinal column that cushions and protects the spine.

Spinal nerve: One of the nerves that originates in the spinal cord.

Spinal stenosis: Narrowing of the open spaces in the spine. This can cause compression of the nerve roots or spinal cord by bony spurs or soft tissues, such as discs, in the spinal canal. This occurs most often in the lumbar spine (in the low back) but also occurs in the cervical spine (in the neck) and less often in the thoracic spine (in the upper back).

Spinal tumor: A tumor located within the spinal column that compresses the nerves of the spine.

Dr. Richard Busch III

Spine: The column of bone known as the vertebral column, which runs down the middle of the back and surrounds and protects the spinal cord. The spine can be categorized according to level of the body: cervical spine (neck), thoracic spine (upper and middle back), and lumbar spine (lower back).

Spinous process: A slender projection from the back of a vertebra, which is where muscles and ligaments are attached.

Spondylitis: Inflammation of one or more of the vertebrae of the spine. Diffuse inflammation of the spine is seen in the disease ankylosing spondylitis. Localized spondylitis is seen with infections of a certain area of the spine, such as in Pott's disease.

Spondylosis: Degeneration of the disc spaces between the vertebrae. This finding in the spine is commonly associated with osteoarthritis.

Subluxation: When one or more bones of the spine move out of position and cause pressure on the nerves.

Surgery: Surgery is the work done by a surgeon. An operation to correct a problem.

Tendon: The tissue that attaches muscle to bone. A tendon is flexible, but also fibrous and tough. When a tendon becomes inflamed, the condition is referred to as tendinitis or tendonitis. Inflamed tendons are at risk for rupture.

TENS: Transcutaneous Electric Neural Stimulator unit, which helps interrupt pain messages to the brain. Developed by C. Norman Shealy, M.D., Ph.D.

Tethers: Imagine that when performing surgery you need to cut through tissue to get to the area you want to affect. This tissue is not just connected in the area that is cut, but can travel throughout the body. When the tissue is sutured or stitched up, this can create a tethering effect that can in essence cause painful symptoms throughout the body.

Tissue meninges: The system of membranes that envelops the central nervous system. The meninges consist of three layers: the dura mater, the arachnoid mater, and the pia mater. The primary function of the meninges and of the cerebrospinal fluid is to protect the central nervous system.

Trauma: Any injury, whether physically or emotionally inflicted. Trauma is a serious or critical bodily injury, wound, or shock. This definition is often associated with trauma medicine practiced in emergency rooms.

Vertebra: A vertebra is one of 33 bony segments that form the spinal column of humans. There are 7 cervical, 12 thoracic, 5 lumbar, 5 sacral (fused into 1 sacrum bone) and 4 coccygeal (fused into 1 coccyx bone).

Vertebrae: The preferred plural of vertebra.

Vessel: A tube in the body that carries fluids: blood vessels or lymph vessels.

X-ray: High-energy radiation with waves shorter than those of visible light. In low doses, X-rays are used for making images that help to diagnose disease, and in high doses to treat cancer.

ANNOTATED BIBLIOGRAPHY

Synopsis of Research on Cervical and Lumbar Decompression/ Traction

Onel D et al. CT investigation of the effects of traction on lumbar herniation. Spine. 1989;14:82-90. Thirty patients with lumbar herniations underwent traction in a CT scanner at >50% body weight for 20 minutes. Herniation retraction occurred in 70% and good clinical improvements were seen in over 93%. The authors concluded improved blood flow was the source of healing and that the traction did not create negative intradiscal pressure due to inadequate traction force.

Tilaro F. *Canadian Journal of Clinical Medicine.* 1998;5:1-7. Decompression therapy significantly reduced intradiscal pressure. Promoting retraction of the herniation, improving diffusion gradient into the disc that allows nutrients and healing.

Note: controversy whether decompression actually occurs and if it occurs how functional is it once the patient stands or sits and weight bearing reoccurs.

Nachemson A. Intradiscal pressure. *Journal of Neurosurgery* 1995;82:1095. Criticized Tilaro experimental setup saying that there wasn't a control group, patients were not randomly assigned, and lacked follow-up scores. Reported the study was not clinically meaningful due to these flaws.

Saal JA, Saal JS. Nonoperative treatment of herniated lumbar disc with radiculopathy (leg pain). *Spine.* 1989;14(4):431-437. Fifty eight subjects; 86% had good-to-excellent results with inclusive conservative program to include traction and trunk stabilization exercises.

Annotated Bibliography

Mathews JA et al. Manipulation and traction for lumbago and sciatica. *Physio Pract.* 1988;4:201. Eight-five percent reported substantial relief with a controlled trial of traction combined with manipulative therapy. Traction force applied at 100 pounds for 20 minutes.

Constatoyannis C et al. Intermittent cervical traction for radiculopathy due to large volume herniations. *Journal of Manipulative and Physiological Therapeutics.* 2002;25(3). Four subjects displayed complete resolution of symptoms after three weeks of cervical traction.

Erhard R et al. Intermittent cervical traction and thoracic manipulation for management of mild cervical compressive myelopathy attributed to cervical herniated disc: A case series. *Journal of Orthopaedic and Sports Physical Therapy.* 2004;34(11). Intermittent cervical traction and manipulation of the thoracic spine was useful for the reduction of pain scores and level of disability in patients with mild cervical compressive myelopathy attributed to herniated disc.

Shealy N, Leroy P. New concepts in back pain management. *AJPM.* 1998;(1)20:239-241. The application of supine lumbar traction altering the angle of pull from 10° to 30° and progression to peak force enhanced distraction at specific levels in the lumbar spine. Increase distraction at L5/S1 with 10° angle of pull and L3 with 30° angle of pull.

Weatherall VF. Comparison of electrical activity in the sacrospinalis musculature during traction in two different positions. *Journal of Orthopaedic and Sports Physical Therapy.* 1995;(8):382-390. EMG electrical activity shown to be similar in the prone versus supine positions.

Letchuman R, Deusinger RH. Comparison of sacrospinalis myoelectric activity and pain levels in patients undergoing static and intermittent lumbar traction. *Spine.* 1993;18(10):1361-1365. Improved comfort and less muscle guarding noted in the intermittent traction group.

Nanno M. Effects of intermittent cervical traction on muscle pain. EMG and flowmetric studies on cervical paraspinals. *Journal of Nippon Medical School*. April 1994;61(2):137-47. Intermittent cervical traction was shown to be effective in relieving pain, improving blood flow and increasing myoelectric signals in the effected muscles.

Chung TS, Lee YJ et al. Reducibility of cervical herniation: Evaluation at MRI during cervical traction with a nonmagnetic device. *Radiology*. December 2002;225(3):895-900. Twenty-nine patients and seven healthy volunteers had intermittent cervical traction while in MR. Substantial increase in vertebral length was seen. Full herniation reduction in three patients and partial reduction in eighteen was reported.

Hseuh TC et al. Evaluation of the effects of pulling angle and force on intermittent cervical traction. *Journal of the Formosan Medical Association*. 1991;90(12):1234-1249. Traction under 30° created longest gap at C4-6 and under 35° created longest gap at C6-T1.

Gionis TA, Groteke E. Spinal decompression. Clinical study evaluating the effect of nonsurgical intervention on symptoms of spine patients with herniated and degenerative disc disease. *Orthopedic Technology Review*. November to December 2003;5(6):36. Of 219 subjects, 86% reported completed resolution of symptoms and 84% of this group remained pain-free for three months.

END NOTES
BY CHAPTER

Chapter 1

(1) Epidemiology and Risk Factors for Spine Pain, *Neurol Clin.* 2007, May,25(2):353-71. Rubin Dl

(2) The Hidden Impact of Musculoskeletal Disorders on Americans, *United State Bone and Joint Initiative*, 2018.

(3) *Adv Anesth. 2010*; 28(1): 269–284, Tiffany L. Tsai, BA, Laura P. Sands, PhD, and Jacqueline M. Leung, MD, MPH

(4) *The Back Letter*, Volume 33, No 5, 2018

(5) Dislocation of a primary total hip arthroplasty is more common in patients with a lumbar spinal fusion, *The Spine Journal*, October 2016, Volume 16, Issue 10, Supplement, Pages S263–S264 Lead author Aaron J. Buckland , MBBS

(6) The Effectiveness and Risks of Fluoroscopically Guided Cervical Transforaminal Injections of Steroids: A Systematic Review with Comprehensive Analysis of the Published Data, *Pain Medicine* 2017; 18: 239-251 Andrew Engel, MD

Also (6)Epidural injections in prevention of surgery for spinal pain: systematic review and meta-analysis of randomized controlled trials, *The Spine Journal*, Vol 15, Iss 2, Feb 2015, , Joshua M.Horowitz, Doab C.Steven, P.Cohen MD

(7) FDA Drug Safety Communication: FDA requires label changes to warn of rare but serious neurologic problems after epidural corticosteroid injections for pain, https://www.fda.gov/Drugs/DrugSafety/ucm394280.htm

(8) Alarming Escalation of Fusion Surgery – What Can be Done?, *American Chiropractic Association*, January 07, 2016, Ron Feise, DC

(9) 15 Facts on Spinal Fusion for Low Back Pain, *US News*, May 29, 2015, Lisa Esposito

(10) Katz JN. Lumbar disc disorders and low-back pain: socioeconomic factors and consequence [review]. *J Bone Joint Surg Am.* 2006;88(suppl 2): 21-24   www.ACAtoday.org/Patients./Health-Wellness-Information/Back-Pain-Fact-and Statistics

Chapter 2

(1) www.ACAtoday.org/Patients./Health-Wellness-Information/Back-Pain-Fact-and Statistics

(2) *Harvard Health Publishing*: Depression and pain; Updated: March 21, 2017, Orig. Published: June, 2009, https://www.health.harvard.edu/mind-and-mood/depression-and-pain

Chapter 3

(1) Effects of Vertebral Axial Decompression of Intervebral Disc, *J Neurosurgery* 81: 350-353, 1994, Dr. Gustavo Ramos and Dr. William Martin

(2) Eliciting the Patient's Agenda- Secondary Analysis of Recorded Clinical Encounters, *Journal of General Internal Medicine*: January 2019, Volume 34, Issue 1, pp 36–40

(3) Variability in diagnostic error rates, *Spine* J, 2017 April 17 (554-561) Herzog R, Elgor DR, Flanders AE, Moley PJ.

(4) The Accuracy of MRI in the Detection of Lumbar Disc Containment, https://www.ncbi.nlm.nih.gov/pmc/articles/PMC2566558/https://www.ncbi.nlm.nih.gov/pmc/articles/PMC2566558, Bradley K Weiner 1,2 and Rikin Patel

Chapter 4

No endnotes.

Chapter 5

(1) CDC Guideline for Prescribing Opioids for Chronic Pain, https://www.cdc.gov/drugoverdose/prescribing/guideline.html , Retrieved 12-20-2018

(2) The Back Letter, *Wolters Kluwer Health*, In Vol. 33, No. 5, 2018

(3) *Int'l Journ. Of Rehabilitation Research,* Lumbar fusion compared with conservative treatment in patients with chronic low back pain: a meta-analysis. March 2014 - Volume 37 - Issue 1 - p 2–8, Saltychev, Mikhaila; Eskola, Merjab; Laimi, Katri

(4) Spine Surgeons Speak Out About Artificial Disc Replacement, *Spine Universe*, Michael Fehlings, MD. Retrieved December 5, 2018

End Notes
Chapter 6

(1)Expert Discusses Living With Chemotherapy-Induced Peripheral Neuropathy, *CURE*, July 24, 2017, Brielle Urciuoli

(2)https://www.foundationforpn.org/what-is-peripheral-neuropathy/types-risk-factors/12-10-18

Chapter 7

(1) Diabetes: Our Nation's Most Expensive Health Condition, *US News.com*, March 28, 2018, William T. Cefalu, M.D., Contributor

(2) CDC https://www.cdc.gov/obesity/data/adult.html

(3) CDC, Prevalence of Both Diagnosed and Undiagnosed Diabetes, https://www.cdc.gov/diabetes/data/statistics-report/diagnosed-undiagnosed.html, 12-11-2018

(4) WEBMD: Peripheral Neuropathy and Diabetes, https://www.webmd.com/diabetes/peripheral-neuropathy-risk-factors-symptoms#1, 12-11-2018

Chapter 8

No end notes

Chapter 9

(1) Accelerated telomere shortening in response to life stress, Proc Natl Acad Sci U S A. 2004 Dec 7;101(49):17312-5. Epub 2004 Dec 1 Epel ES1, Blackburn EH, Lin J, Dhabhar FS, Adler NE, Morrow JD, Cawthon RM.

(2) A Clinical Study of Visualization on Depressed White Blood Cell Count in Medical Patients, *Applied Psychophysiology and Biofeedback* 25(2):117-28 · July 2000, Vann Williams Donaldson

Chapter 10

(1) Risk of vertebrobasilar stroke and chiropractic care: results of a population-based case-control and case-crossover study, *Journal of Manipulative and Physiological Therapeutics*, Cassidy JD, Boyle E, Côté P, et al., 2009

(2) Better memory functioning associated with higher total and low-density lipoprotein cholesterol levels in very elderly subjects without the apolipoprotein e4 allele, *Am J Geriatric Psychiatry*, 2008, Sep16.

ABOUT THE AUTHOR

Dr. Richard E. Busch III has been nationally recognized for his nonsurgical approach to back and neck pain. Even amid today's medical culture of drugs and surgery, he worked to develop the DRS Protocol™ for back and neck pain, the Busch Neuropathy Protocol™, the Busch Knee Protocol™ – all noninvasive, drug-free treatments that have successful, proven results. He believed that patients deserved better and has proven that patients can get the relief they need without enduring endless cycles of frustration with more invasive and less effective methods. There is no reason for anyone to spend another day, week or month in pain.

Dr. Richard Busch III

CPSIA information can be obtained
at www.ICGtesting.com
Printed in the USA
BVHW011555190622
639756BV00001B/2